Equine-Facilitated Psychotherapy and Learning

Equine-Facilitated Psychotherapy and Learning

The Human-Equine Relational Development (HERD) Approach

Veronica Lac, PhD
Executive Director, The HERD Institute,
New Albany, OH, United States

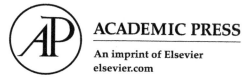

ACADEMIC PRESS

An imprint of Elsevier
elsevier.com

⎿c Press is an imprint of Elsevier
⎿ondon Wall, London EC2Y 5AS, United Kingdom
⎿25 B Street, Suite 1800, San Diego, CA 92101-4495, United States
50 Hampshire Street, 5th Floor, Cambridge, MA 02139, United States
The Boulevard, Langford Lane, Kidlington, Oxford OX5 1GB, United Kingdom

Notices

Knowledge and best practice in this field are constantly changing. As new research and experience broaden our understanding, changes in research methods, professional practices, or medical treatment may become necessary.

Practitioners and researchers must always rely on their own experience and knowledge in evaluating and using any information, methods, compounds, or experiments described herein. In using such information or methods they should be mindful of their own safety and the safety of others, including parties for whom they have a professional responsibility.

To the fullest extent of the law, neither the Publisher nor the authors, contributors, or editors, assume any liability for any injury and/or damage to persons or property as a matter of products liability, negligence or otherwise, or from any use or operation of any methods, products, instructions, or ideas contained in the material herein.

British Library Cataloguing-in-Publication Data
A catalogue record for this book is available from the British Library

Library of Congress Cataloging-in-Publication Data
A catalog record for this book is available from the Library of Congress

ISBN: 978-0-12-812601-1

For Information on all Academic Press publications
visit our website at https://www.elsevier.com/books-and-journals

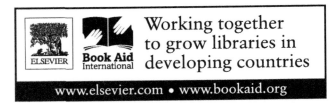

Working together
to grow libraries in
developing countries

www.elsevier.com • www.bookaid.org

Publisher: Nikki Levy
Acquisition Editor: Dennis McGonagle
Editorial Project Manager: Sarah Jane Watson
Senior Production Project Manager: Priya Kumaraguruparan
Cover Designer: Mark Rogers

Typeset by MPS Limited, Chennai, India

For Rupert, the Goth rock pony that stole my heart and set me on this journey of equine discovery. You are in my heart always, and I am forever grateful to the lessons you offered me. I hope your days are spent running free in green pastures, wherever you may be.

Contents

About the Author   xi
Contributors   xiii
Foreword   xv
Acknowledgments   xvii

Part I

1. Introduction   3

2. Why Horses? What is Equine Therapy?   7

    The Therapeutic Benefits of the Human–Equine Bond in
        Equine-Assisted Interventions   9
    "Equine Therapy": The Need for Clarification   10
    Therapy Versus Therapeutic   10
    Therapeutic Riding   11
    The HERD Institute Model of EFL   13
    Equine-Assisted/Facilitated Therapy   13
    What Is Equine-Assisted/Facilitated Psychotherapy?   14
    Differing Modalities in EFMHS   14
    The HERD Institute Model of EFP   16

3. Philosophical Foundations   17

    Philosophical Relevance   17
    Human Animals   18
    Phenomenology and Embodiment   19
    EFPL and Phenomenology   21
    Buber's *I-Thou*   22
    Embodied Connections of Phenomenology and *I-Thou*   25
    Buber's *I-Thou* and Horses   25
    Discovery of *I-It* Encounters   26

4. Theoretical Foundations   27

    Broadening Horizons and Digging Deep   27
    Core Theory   27
    Here and Now   28
    What and How   29

I-Thou   31
Lost in Translation   32
Embodiment and Authenticity   32
The Embodied Relational Self   33

**5. Theoretical Foundations II: Where Does the
     Horse Fit in?**   35

The Magic of Horses   35
Projection/Mirroring   37
Attachment   39
Groundwork   39
A Word About Working With Trauma   40
Mounted Work   40

Part II

6. Ethical Practice in EFPL   45
Veronica Lac and Elisabeth Crabtree

The Professional Relationship   46
Confidentiality   47
Client Safety   47
Continued Development   48
Discussion on Safety and Ethics   48
The HERD Safety Protocol   48
Safety Around Horses   48
A Safe Therapeutic Relationship   50
The Role of Assistants   51
Cofacilitator   51
Equine Support Staff   51
Adjuvants   51
A Safe Place   52
Leveling the Playing Field: A Place in the Herd   53
Ethics of Working With Horses   55
Horsemanship Development   57
Horse Suitability   57

7. The HERD Model of Equine-Facilitated Psychotherapy 61

Stage One: Sharing Space   61
Stage Two: Release and Expand   63
Stage Three: Deepening   66
Stage Four: Coming Home   67
Stage Five: Integration   68
Summary   70

8. The HERD Model of Equine Facilitated Learning   71

    Scope of Practice   71
    The HERD Model of EFL   72
    Stage One: Meeting   73
    Experiential Learning   76
    Meeting the Horses   78
    Stage Two: Relating   79
    Stage Three: Integrating   80
    Themes, Culture, and Language   81
    Summary   82

9. The HERD Model of EFP in Action   85

    You Had Me at Hello   86
    New Beginnings: Taking the First Step   88
    Case Studies   90
    Case Study 1: Amy's Story   90
    Release and Expand   92
    Revisiting the Lessons Learned   95
    Back and Forth   95
    Case Study 2: Embodied Touch   97
    Case Study 3: The Language of Love   102
    Case Study 4: One Breath, One Movement   107
    Case Study 5: Integrating the HERD Model of EFP With
        Humanistic Play Therapy   114
    What Is Humanistic Play Therapy?   114
    Case Study 6: Sinking into Support   118
    Case Study 7: We Are All Connected   121
    Case Study 8: Working With Veterans   127
    Conclusion   131

10. The HERD Model of EFL in Action   133

    Case Study 1: Creating a "ME"-Shaped Space   134
    Case Study 2: A Bubble of Two   138
    Case Study 3: Anticipating Needs   142
    Case Study 4: Everyone Wants to Belong   148
    Case Study 5: Resilience and Vulnerability   151
    Case Study 6: Just Sniff   154
    Conclusion   157

Part III

11. Horse Sense, Business Sense   161

    Starting Equine-Facilitated Work   161
    Setting Up Shop   161
    Preparing Yourself   161

Human First Aid Kit 164
Equine First Aid Kit 164
Where Are You Going to Do the Work? 165
Facilities 165
The Human-Equine Relationship Continuum 165
Business Arrangements 167
Managing the Space 169
Advocates 169
Clients 169
Fee Structure 170
Networking and Marketing 170
Demonstrations and Workshops 171
Conclusion 171

12. **Final Words** 173

Bibliography 177
Index 181

About the Author

Veronica Lac, PhD. LPC
Dr. Veronica Lac has 20 years of experience as a corporate trainer and mental health professional as well as a certified therapeutic riding instructor, providing her with an integrated perspective to EFPL. Her academic background includes a Masters in Training and Performance Management, a Masters in Gestalt Psychotherapy, and a PhD in Psychology. She is trained in a number of models in EFPL including a mentorship in Adventures in Awareness with Barbara Rector, a pioneering influence in this field, and certification through the Gestalt Equine Institute of the Rockies. This has allowed her to combine her theoretical understanding into a relational and embodied approach to EFPL. Veronica is passionate about working with clients to enable them to reach their full potential, and is an experienced corporate trainer offering one-to-one coaching and organizational consultancy. Clients range from large corporate businesses to individuals, couples, and families.

Veronica was a UKCP Registered Psychotherapist in the United Kingdom, and since moving to the United States in 2011, she has gained licensure as a professional counselor and completed her PhD in Psychology through Saybrook University. She specializes in working with eating disorders, trauma, and attachment and has developed equine and canine assisted programs for at-risk adolescents in collaboration with residential treatment centers and eating disorder clinics. She is also a PATH registered therapeutic riding instructor for clients with cognitive, physical, and emotional disabilities. Veronica is passionate about research in the field of equine facilitated psychotherapy and has multiple publications internationally in peer-reviewed journals.

Contributors

Elisabeth Crabtree MSc., GEP, MIAEB, AISRB

In addition to a long career as a Business and Management Consultant, Elisabeth also has extensive teaching experience at colleges and universities. Elisabeth combines her life-long horsemanship skills with her business experience in order to develop equine-facilitated programs. She works with individuals and groups, with an emphasis on professional and business development, communication skills, and team building. A lifelong equestrian, Elisabeth is certified through the Gestalt Equine Institute of the Rockies in Gestalt Equine Psychotherapy (GEP), holds an OK Corral Series certification in Equine Assisted Psychotherapy (EAP) and Equine Assisted Learning (EAL) as well as a Masters in Education and Training. She is an official coach with the International Society of Rider Biomechanics, a founding member of the International Association of Equestrian Biomechanics, and a Certified Equine First Aid Instructor through Equi-Health Canada, all of which supports her somatically based approach to EFPL.

Chris Goodall, LISW-S

Chris is a licensed independent Social Work Supervisor, certified by the equine assisted growth and learning association as both a mental health professional and an equine specialist and a member of the Professional Association of Therapeutic Horsemanship International. She has worked in community based, inpatient, and residential behavioral health settings. Chris is currently employed by the Louis Stokes Cleveland DVAMC working in the Psychosocial Rehabilitation and Recovery Center where she initiated an equine-facilitated psychotherapy program. Chris is a lecturer for Lake Erie College for the Equine Facilitated Psychotherapy and Learning program, and is in private practice offering both traditional and equine-facilitated psychotherapy services.

Foreword

Dr. Veronica Lac offers us a clear view of the future in this practical concise treatise on practice and teaching wellness work with horses. It has been a personal privilege for me to learn from mentor and work with this gifted professional. This volume contains illuminating answers for those interested in offering services with the help of horses in the fields of psychotherapy and experiential education.

A remarkably clear and practical conceptual framework for practice of Equine Facilitated Psychotherapy and teaching of Equine Facilitated Learning (EFP/EFL), Veronica's book offers the reader specific examples of various elements of the Human-Equine Relational Development (HERD) model. Developed by Veronica over the course of her international studies, PhD research, and practice with horses helping people, this powerful and well thought out process for engaging people relationally with horses to experience and embody the gifts horses offer to humans is the new wave of the future. Veronica is a certified PATH Int. instructor, and this experience adds considerably to the depth and variety of her skill base. The case studies offer a powerful insight into the HERD model in action.

I first met Veronica in 2013 at the European Horse Assisted Education Conference in Cleveland, and then again at the 2015 PATH Intl. Conference where she and her practice partner, Elisabeth Crabtree, offered an eye opening session on the wide varieties and forms possible when two imaginative and well-trained professionals collaborate and design potent individualized sessions for their clients. These two focused on relational aspects of learning to befriend horses safely while encouraging their clients to test their personal edges and grow. These ethical and relational principles are evident throughout this book.

In this volume, Veronica includes her colleague Elisabeth's contributions in an illuminating chapter on staffing and facility considerations. Another colleague, Chris Goodall, contributes a skilled chapter on considerations and suggestions for working with Veterans in EFPL groups. Veronica also covers the enhanced potential of working experientially with teams of people from the corporate and business world.

YES, it is true, I am very partial to the organic approach of listening and allowing the horses to express their immense talent to fully bloom in an environment of a well thought out safety protocol, precise preparation and collaboration with staff both two and four legged. Prepare for a truly inspiring read that is sure to pique your own co-creative gifts as you listen and learn with your herd.

Heart Hugs,
Barbara K. Rector, MA
Skyview Casita, Tucson, AZ, United States
January 2, 2017

Acknowledgments

First and foremost, to my husband, Quan, I offer my deepest gratitude. For 20 years, he has stood by my side as I have tumbled from one obsession to the next, daydreaming my way through my life, looking for an elusive calling that would fill my soul. Instead of offering me pragmatic advice, he offered me his unwavering love, support, and encouragement to venture beyond my immediate horizon, and to follow my heart toward the path which intuitively felt right. It is because of his belief in me that my day-dreams can become reality. For all the sacrifices that this took, the emotional roller coaster, time, and finances, I am enormously grateful. The HERD Institute, and this book would not exist without his belief in me. These achievements are not mine alone but shared in equal measure with him.

Duey Freeman and Joan Rieger, at the Gestalt Equine Institute of the Rockies where I began my training in EFP, were instrumental in instilling the belief that this work is powerful and life changing when we place the relationship at the heart of the work. It was here at GEIR that I first experienced the magic of the coming together of horse and human herds that has been so influential in my development as a practitioner.

I am thankful for the time I spent in Arizona with Barbara Rector and Anna Calek. Their belief in me as a practitioner and teacher, and their encouragement, provided the impetus I needed to create The HERD Institute and write this book. Barbara's mentorship reaffirmed for me to trust my intuition with my horses as well as to trust them to guide me in our joint endeavors.

I will forever be indebted to my childhood friend and sister, Lisa Clark, not only for infecting me with her love of horses, but equally importantly, for sharing her family with me, particularly, Elisabeth (Lis) Crabtree, for almost 30 years. I have had the joy of sharing my GEIR journey with Lis. Our conversations about coming into this work from opposite tracks have been crucial in developing my way of working with horses. Lis has been there for me throughout the years, no matter what, and wherever life has taken me. Knowing that she will always have my back has given me the confidence to challenge and step beyond the boundaries that I would otherwise have been restricted by. It is an honor to call her a friend and colleague.

Louis Hoffman has been the most dedicated teacher I have ever known. I am thankful for his exacting requirements, compassionate feedback, and invitations to participate and collaborate on presentations, papers, and conferences. His faith in my abilities has opened doors I never imagined possible.

I have been humbled by all my clients, past and present, for sharing their journeys with me and allowing me to walk with them for a while. They have all enormously contributed to my personal and clinical development. Without their openness and willingness to sink deeper into their reflections, this book would not have been possible.

Finally, I am beyond grateful for all the animals in my life who inspire me to do this work. To our dog, Alfie, whose presence initially alerted me to the power of the human animal bond, and whose loyal companionship has seen me through my darkest days and warmed my heart with every beat of his, I offer my continued devotion. To Tyson, who reaffirms my faith that love can change anything. To my equine herds, past and present, I profess my heartfelt gratitude: Rupert, Reba, Cheyenne, Arrow, Infinity, Tess, Lucinda, Spirit, Samson, Freeman, Isaac, and Dina; I thank them all for leading me home.

Part I

Chapter 1

Introduction

The field of equine-assisted/facilitated psychotherapy (EAP/EFP) and equine-facilitated learning (EFL) is beginning to gain popularity in North America and Europe. There have been a number of publications recently that have made major contributions to the field in terms of theory and practice, outlining ways to work with differing populations, and offering practical suggestions in terms of exercises to set up with clients.

As a growing modality, there is still much to do in terms of empirical research and explication of theories. As yet, there is little available in the way of solid philosophical foundations from a scholarly perspective of the work. This book is an attempt to open up the dialogue for both scholars and practitioners to collectively build upon the work of the pioneers in our field. It takes a deeper look at the philosophy behind what we mean when we say that EAP/EFP and EFL helps to build relationships. Whether we are working with therapy clients—individuals, couples, families, and groups—or in educational or corporate/organizational environments, it is important to understand our philosophical origins in order to bring the theory alive in our practice. This book is for students, licensed mental health practitioners, educators, and corporate/organizational trainers who are interested in incorporating horses into their work with clients, as well as for those who are already out there offering equine-facilitated learning and therapeutic interventions. It is for the academic scholar wanting to delve deeper into the philosophical origins of this field, as well as those who are new to the language of philosophy.

The Human-Equine Relational Development (HERD) Institute offers training and development for Equine-Facilitated Psychotherapy and Learning (EFPL) practitioners. The approach is influenced by my years of experience in practice, and the HERD approach to EFPL is the result of my doctoral research. This book also serves as the core text for the training at the HERD Institute. The HERD Institute aims to create a global community, of students and practitioners for EFPL who are committed to furthering the work of the pioneers of our field. We offer an inclusive environment, embracing an attitude of abundance, and honor the potential of all our members. We aim for EFPL to be recognized as an empirically based treatment and educational modality, and support members to develop the integrity of their personal philosophy, expand their knowledge and skills, and broaden their horizons

Equine-Facilitated Psychotherapy and Learning. DOI: http://dx.doi.org/10.1016/B978-0-12-812601-1.00001-8

through continuous learning and practice. Our core values are centered on a passion for learning, compassion for our fellow beings, and the commitment to professional and personal development. It is my hope that these values are evident throughout this book.

My experience in the last 20 years as a corporate trainer and mental health professional, as well as a certified therapeutic riding instructor, provides me with an integrated perspective to EFPL. My academic background includes a masters in training and performance management, a masters in gestalt psychotherapy, and a PhD in psychology. I have trained in a number of models in EFP/EFL including a mentorship in adventures in awareness with Barbara Rector, a pioneering influence in this field, and certification through the Gestalt Equine Institute of the Rockies. This has allowed me to integrate my theoretical understanding into a somatically based clinical practice and training methodology. The theoretical basis for the HERD approach to EFPL is a synthesis of existential-humanistic psychology, gestalt psychotherapy, therapeutic riding principles, and somatically based experiential learning.

Body language and nonverbal communication have always intrigued me. Within the corporate world, many decision-making moments can be observed through subtle shifts in body language and nonverbal cues. Working as a corporate trainer to senior executives in a wide range of businesses allowed me to sink deeper into the nonverbal culture of organizations. Throughout my training and practice as a gestalt therapist, I have been particularly impacted by how much information is available through paying attention to both my client's, and my own, body process. From mindfully breathing and moving exercises, to explorations of body positioning and postures, I have gained a deeper insight into the embodied relational process of therapy.

Not long after graduating from my gestalt masters' program, I decided to treat myself to a block of horseback riding lessons. Around the same time, my husband and I decided to bring a puppy into our lives. The combination of these two events shifted my professional focus to the potential of animal facilitated therapy and learning, and consequently an even fuller immersion into embodiment-based practice. In my clinical work, I have specialized in working with eating disorders, trauma, and attachment and have developed equine and canine facilitated programs for at-risk adolescents in collaboration with residential treatment centers, eating disorder clinics, and intensive familiy-based out-patient programs. As a PATH International registered therapeutic riding instructor, I work with clients with cognitive, physical, and emotional challenges. As a corporate trainer, I have worked with the CEOs and board level directors of Fortune 500 companies internationally in equine-faciliated learning sessions.

Ultimately, when we are with animals, my academic credentials are irrelevant. Presence is priority. As an animal lover, I am often more comfortable in the company of my dogs and horses than with people, and it is from them that I have learned the most about embodied presence. Over time, I began to inhabit myself more fully bodily; became more attentive to energetic presence within myself and of others; found fluidity of intention through breath and movement; and heightened my awareness of how I block my own energetic process. Most of all, I discovered the depth of relationship that can be reached when I fully embody each moment.

As I reflect on my motivation to do this work and write this book, I have come to realize what the horses have always known. The most meaningful learning does not come from techniques or knowledge. As therapists, educators, trainers, and coaches, we bring ourselves fully into the moment and engage in relationships with our clients as fellow human beings. We share the moment, the space, and the air that we breathe as we connect with our clients and ourselves. There is mutuality in this connection that allows us to be not just a professional, but a living, breathing, sentient being with them. It is in this togetherness that healing and growth occurs. As our clients find their place in the world, in their "herd," in their lives, we too find ourselves. This interconnectedness allows us to take ownership of the fact that our every action, or inaction, creates a ripple effect for those around us. Much like horses in a herd, we cannot help but to make an impact on each other. So what draws me towards offering the HERD approach for EFPL, and doing this work, is the same as what helps us all to find meaning: connection, relationship, and knowing that our existence matters.

Chapter 2

Why Horses? What is Equine Therapy?

Arriving at the barn one day, I pulled up to the parking lot adjacent to the large paddock where the mares are usually turned out. As I got out of my truck, I noticed that all the mares were milling around near the gate. I spotted my mare, Reba, who had started pacing the fence line upon seeing me and was whinnying loudly. Although this was unusual, I thought she was simply waiting to be brought in for her morning grain and was telling me to hurry up, so I continued into the barn to fetch her halter. As I walked back towards the paddock, Reba became more frantic. I noticed that one of the mares was facing the opposite way to the rest of the herd and appeared to be exceptionally close to the four-board fencing. Then, I caught a glimpse of metal flashing in the sunlight along the fence and realized that the mare had somehow got her back leg stuck on the top rail. Her hoof was caught by the top of her shoe, on top of the wooden fence. Reaching for my phone, I called our barn owner as I ran towards the paddock. Sizing up the situation, I realized that there was no way that I could free the mare without taking the fence board off. I had to wait for help.

I walked into the paddock and the horses parted to make way for me to get to the injured mare, Lady. She was sweating and shaking. I had no idea how long she had been there. I stood with her and stroked her neck to reassure her that help was on its way. Within a couple of minutes, Carrie, the barn owner was at the fence with a hammer. I wanted to make sure that Lady didn't fall over as soon as she got free, so I put Reba's halter on her as Carrie pried the fence rail off the post and lifted her leg free. She stumbled forward a couple of steps before regaining her balance and exhaled.

The rest of the mares had stayed nearby. As I led Lady towards the gate, each one of her companions came up to her and they sniffed at each other. The first one to come over was the lead mare in the herd. She placed her muzzle on Lady's withers and rubbed her lips across her back. Then came Reba, her closest companion. Reba sniffed Lady's neck and down her back towards the hind leg that had been stuck. She paused as she made her way back up to her hip, and breathed out. Lady turned her head

Equine-Facilitated Psychotherapy and Learning. DOI: http://dx.doi.org/10.1016/B978-0-12-812601-1.00002-X

7

as if to acknowledge Reba's concern, and exhaled deeply. I was moved to tears as I watched them connecting, and in my mind at least, reassuring each other that everything would now be okay. Panic over. Peace and harmony restored.

As I handed the mare over to Carrie, who had by then called the vet who was on his way, I turned to Reba who was standing by my side. "Thank you, for letting me help your friend. And thank you for trying to get my attention."

The Human Equine Relational Development (HERD) approach is based on the understanding that both humans and horses are sentient beings. Our shared evolution over millennia has provided us with the ability to connect across species in a deep and profound way. This can only happen, of course, if we listen closely to ourselves, and our equine partners, through a compassionate and authentic way of relating. In developing our relational capacity with our horses, we can come to a deeper understanding of ourselves. In turn, we can transfer this way of being-in-the-world into other areas of our lives and relationships. The human—equine relationship is historically central in the mythical and spiritual tales of many cultures around the world. Our coexistence over the centuries has instilled a sense of awe and wonder at these majestic creatures, and it is with reverence and respect that we step into their world to invite them to partner with us in the work that we do. The HERD philosophy is one of compassion, present moment awareness, and connection. It is an embodied relational journey that honors our equine partners and their way of being.

Horses embody the concept of relationship, living in the present moment with the whole of their being. As herd animals, they survive through their ability to be constantly aware of their surroundings and each other. Archeologist K.A. Oma believes that in the presence of humans, horses will transfer their herd-based relational instincts to people, including viewing people as part of their herd:

> The human—horse relationship is founded on interconnectedness where a joint participation in the world leads to a state of humans and horses being mixed. Inherently, species that live together come to attune to each other, and a platform of communication based upon sympathetic responses to each other is established.

Horses and humans have co-evolved for millennia, as evidenced by the cave paintings in France dating back to 30,000 B.C., and have been woven into the fabric of human lives through being a source of transportation, power for machinery, war heroes, and companions. Horses have been depicted in mythologies, fairy tales, and legends as metaphors for strength, courage, resilience, and compassion. From the ancient Greeks and Egyptians, to the Chinese Dynasties and Mongolian shamans, humans have turned to the horse for their wisdom and guidance. According to Hamilton, author of

Evidence-Based Horsemanship, the relationship between horses and humans allows for the unique opportunity to switch off left-brain thinking, and instead "return to a primal, nonverbal state of awareness." Without the interference of language, we reconnect with the energy shared among all life forms. The connection is palpable and immediate.

There is no greater example of this attunement than between horse and rider, as Oma points out: "when the human and the horse are in tune together, the relationship is what matters, and species are forgotten." Riding is an act of partnership; it is a dance and requires trust, fluidity, and whole-hearted presence from both beings. The seamless movements that come from experiencing the feeling of inhabiting each other in an embodied way are crucial to this dance and impact the emotional state of both horse and human.

The HeartMath Institute conducted various studies related to Heart Rate Variability (HRV), which are heart rhythm patterns that correlate to emotional states and can be measured as electromagnetic pulses. The heart generates the body's strongest electromagnetic field, almost 60 times greater than that produced by the brain. Initial studies showed that:

> Negative emotions, such as anger or frustration, are associated with an erratic, disordered, *incoherent* pattern in the heart's rhythms. In contrast, positive emotions, such as love or appreciation, are associated with a smooth, ordered, *coherent* pattern... More specifically, we have demonstrated that sustained positive emotions appear to give rise to a distinct mode of functioning, which we call psychophysiological coherence.

The HeartMath Institute extended their HRV research to horse–human relationships and found that horses' ability to remain coherent to their own emotional states allows them to increase the capacity for human beings to regulate their emotions and achieve psychophysiological coherence in themselves. Of even more significance is that in situations where the horse is relaxed and the human is stressed, the horse's calming energy may be transferred to the person to support them to relax. Additionally, it seems that the state of the horses had a greater influence on the humans than the other way around. This is clear physiological evidence of the horse–human bond, which when applied in a therapeutic context can allow for profound healing.

THE THERAPEUTIC BENEFITS OF THE HUMAN–EQUINE BOND IN EQUINE-ASSISTED INTERVENTIONS

Equine-Assisted Therapy and Learning is an umbrella term that has been used to cover a host of different types of programs that involve the participation of horses for human benefit. There are four categories under this umbrella: (1) Therapeutic Horsemanship, (2) Mental Health, (3) Education, and (4) Organizational. Within these categories lie a milieu of approaches, theories, and practices; some of these are quite distinct from each other, but many of them have shared histories, aims, and blurred boundaries. Furthermore, there is confusion within the field in terms of definitions and a general misunderstanding of the terminology of Equine-Assisted Therapies (EAT).

"EQUINE THERAPY": THE NEED FOR CLARIFICATION

There is much confusion as to what constitutes Equine-Assisted Therapy (EAT), Equine-Assisted Learning (EAL), Equine-Facilitated Psychotherapy (EFP), and Equine-Facilitated Learning (EFL). There have been a growing number of research studies on the efficacy of integrating equines into working within mental health, educational, and organizational settings but there is an inconsistency in the terminologies used to define the work. Specifically, there is confusion amongst both the public and practitioners on what is considered "therapy." Conversationally, the terms "equine therapy" or "equine-assisted learning" are used to denote a wide range of services including, but not limited to, therapeutic riding for children on the autism spectrum, working with Veterans with PTSD, mental health provisions with the inclusion of horses, and teambuilding and leadership training. It is, therefore, crucial to be clear about what services we, as practitioners, are offering and to use the correct terminology with clients who approach us about our services. This is particularly important if you work in an area where licensure and/or professional registrations are required. Precise terminology will not only ensure that your clients know what to expect but will also help you to avoid any legal pitfalls.

THERAPY VERSUS THERAPEUTIC

There are many organizations, both in the United States and in the United Kingdom, where the term "equine therapy" is a catch all term that is used to incorporate horses into various programs. Some of these are nonprofit organizations that focus on therapeutic riding that also offer programs that do not involve horseback riding. These programs are often referred to as EAT or EAL, but are not run by licensed professionals (counselors, social workers, psychologists, or speech, physical, and occupational therapists). There is no doubt that these services are therapeutic for the participants, but they do not qualify as "therapy" (as understood in terms of psychotherapy, speech, physical, and occupational). There are many programs that are staffed predominantly by volunteers, and whilst they may bring a wealth of experience and work with the different populations that utilize the services, they may not be licensed practitioners. An example of this type of program might be hospitals or elderly care homes allowing miniature horses onto the premises for petting, grooming, and companionship. Other programs may be led by trained professionals and supplemented with volunteers. The list below shows examples of the type of programs and interventions that fall into this category:

- Therapeutic Riding
- Community Groups visiting a barn for horse—human interactions (e.g., Alzheimer's patients who benefit from grooming a horse)
- Educational programs visiting a barn for horse—human interactions and learning (e.g., Students with Autism engaging in structured activities with horses to learn about social interactions)
- Special Needs Summer Camps
- Veteran or Prison programs that focus on horsemanship and riding skills only.

Therapeutic riding is a discipline in its own right and will be discussed later, however, the other examples in the list (which is by no means exhaustive) are examples of therapeutic activities that fall under the banner of Equine-Assisted/Facilitated Learning. These are programs that incorporate the therapeutic benefits of being with horses as a way to improve cognitive, physical, and social challenges. Research has shown that simply being in the presence of horses can help participants focus more clearly, engage in social interactions more readily, and improve communication skills.

In addition to the programs listed above, equine-facilitated learning may also incorporate learning with horses in the context of corporate training and/or coaching. These activities utilize the relational and herd dynamics of being in proximity to horses as a way to develop leadership, teambuilding, assertiveness, and communication skills. This is currently a growing area within the field, as the corporate world begins to acknowledge the benefits of bringing employees outside of their office setting and into an experiential learning environment.

Therapeutic Riding

The North American Riding for the Handicapped Association (NAHRA) was founded in 1969 to promote and regulate EAT practices, primarily serving individuals with physical and cognitive disabilities. It has since developed into the Professional Association of Therapeutic Horsemanship International, more commonly referred to as PATH Intl, and is now a leading force in the field of EAT. With over 4000 certified instructors and equine specialists, and around 850 accredited centers around the world, PATH Intl programs offer services to children and adults with physical, emotional, and cognitive challenges through EAT.

Therapeutic horsemanship encompasses the disciplines of hippotherapy and therapeutic riding. Hippotherapy is therapy with the inclusion of the use of horses by licensed physical, speech, or occupational therapists and utilizes the movement of the horse for the benefit of the patient. Therapeutic riding involves teaching individuals with special needs the skills of horseback riding. The fundamental difference in these two disciplines is that hippotherapy requires the involvement of a medical practitioner, whilst therapeutic riding does not. Although the therapeutic riding instructor might also work within a multidisciplinary team that includes occupational, physical, and/or speech therapists, the therapists do not need to be present during the lessons. However, there are similarities in terms of the benefits that clients receive during hippotherapy sessions that are present during therapeutic riding lessons. Additionally, in both of these endeavors, the client works with a team consisting of the instructor or therapist, a horse, and a group of volunteers. The trained volunteers are present to conduct specific tasks such as horse grooming, tacking, leading, and/or side-walking during lessons. Side-walkers walk alongside the horse and rider and are responsible for the safety of the child whilst mounted and on the ground; they also help to engage the children in activities during the lesson.

Benefits of Therapeutic Riding

Therapeutic riding offers an embodied multisensory experience that affects the client's sensory, neurological, psychological, and social processing patterns. Horseback riding focuses on communication between horse and rider both verbally and nonverbally through body positioning. During a therapeutic riding lesson, beginning clients are taught how to ask their horses to walk, halt, and turn. This engages the use of verbal commands as well as body cues that incorporate the movement of seat, legs, and hands. Horseback riding improves balance and core strength, as well as fitness and endurance. Sitting on the horse and staying balanced requires the use of core muscles. As riders progress pass the basic walk, halt, and turns, they are taught to ask their horses to trot. At different gaits, the horse provides different movement patterns and sensory input to the rider. This is particularly beneficial for clients who have difficulties with core stability, gross motor coordination, and balance.

Research into the benefits of therapeutic riding has been somewhat scarce. There also seems to be confusion with terminology, with some studies using the terms therapeutic riding and hippotherapy interchangeably. There is consensus within the research to support the claims that therapeutic riding is beneficial for the special needs population, and particularly for clients diagnosed with autism and Attention-Deficit Hyperactivity Disorder (ADHD). Benefits include improving behavioral issues, quality of life, and motor performance, as well as significant improvements on measures of self-regulation, adaptive expressive language skills, motor skills, and verbal praxis/motor planning skills after as few as 10 weekly lessons.

THE HERD INSTITUTE MODEL OF EFL

At the HERD Institute, we combine the skills, knowledge, and principles of EFL and Therapeutic Riding to offer a powerful model for facilitation in the corporate and educational environment. We firmly believe in practitioners staying within their scope of practice and advocate for a clear distinction between EFL and EFP. It is not enough to simply acknowledge the differences in terminology. It is vital that students and practitioners understand the boundaries between what is "learning" and what is "therapy." Within the HERD Institute Model, this boundary is strongly emphasized, and for that reason, we offer certifications for EFL and EFP as two distinct training programs. Knowing that there is a boundary is not sufficient for EFL practitioners; the skill is in recognizing how to facilitate a session within the safe confines of that boundary, and still work with clients in a deep and meaningful way. We believe that the facilitation skills required for EFL are significantly different to those needed within EFP. We will discuss this in more detail later.

EQUINE-ASSISTED/FACILITATED THERAPY

The "therapy" in EA/FT refers to any type of certified professional therapist, including physical, occupational, speech, and mental health practitioners licensed or certified in psychology, psychotherapy, social work, and counseling. Within the context of counseling, Chandler, an expert in Animal-Assisted Therapy (AAT), offered the following definition:

> A therapist can incorporate the animal into whatever professional style of therapy the therapist already enacts. AAT can be directive or nondirective in its approach. AAT sessions can be integrated into individual or group therapy... AAT is a practice modality and not an independent profession. Persons guiding AAT must have the proper training and credentials for their professional practice, such as those for a licensed professional counselor.

In contrast to Chandler's view that AAT acts as an adjunct to existing therapy, Bar-On, Shapiro, and Gendelman, leaders in Animal-Assisted Psychotherapy argued that AAT not only needs to be acknowledged as an independent profession, but accepted as a form of psychotherapy in its own right. They assert that AAT should not be an adjunct to traditional talking therapies, as incorporating animals into the psychotherapy setting requires additional skills compared to those needed within a human—human therapy relationship. Furthermore, it is important to acknowledge the complex dynamics involved within an AAT session as the relationships include client and animal, client and therapist, therapist and animal, and if working with more than one animal, it also needs to include animal and animal. So it is imperative that the therapist is not only credentialed in his/her own field of expertise but also possess:

> ...extensive knowledge and understanding in the field of animal behavior, animal welfare, and the various levels of the human–animal relationship. One must be skilled in the ways of the unique integration of animals in the therapeutic encounter between man and animals, in a manner that contributes to the therapeutic contact but maintains the animal's welfare.

WHAT IS EQUINE-ASSISTED/FACILITATED PSYCHOTHERAPY?

The inclusion of horses as part of the therapeutic encounter is a relatively new development in the fields of counseling and psychotherapy. There are differing approaches, belief systems, methods, and acronyms that describe and define what, how, and why this is a valuable process for different populations. Equine-Facilitated Psychotherapy (EFP) and Equine-Assisted Psychotherapy (EAP) used, sometimes interchangeably, to refer to this process. There are, of course, distinctions between these approaches, but ultimately, they are based on the fundamental belief that healing, learning, and personal growth and development can be brought about through interacting with horses. These modalities are sometimes referred to collectively as Equine-Facilitated Mental Health Services (EFMHS).

Differing Modalities in EFMHS

Lief Hallberg, author of *The Way of the Horse*, researched the different modalities from which mental health practitioners operated and discovered that practitioners were trained in a variety of theoretical approaches to counseling and psychotherapy; however, regardless of their approach, there was one common thread that ran through all of them, which is the belief that change is most likely to occur through translating insight into action by the experiencing of new situations.

This is the essence of the experiential learning process instilled by Barbara Rector, a pioneer in the field of EFMHS. Rector emphasized that one of the basic principles of incorporating horses into any therapeutic process is the experiential learning that can occur if we "step back, ask the horse, and allow the process to unfold." It is believed that this leads to the development of personal insight for the client. This experiential element is at the core of all EFMHS work. However, there are also many differences, which Hallberg sought to identify in her research, concluding that the two main branches of EFMHS could be summarized through the differences between EAP and EFP.

EAP Versus EFP

While the terms Equine-Assisted Psychotherapy (EAP) and Equine-Facilitated Psychotherapy (EFP) are often used interchangeably, I believe that there is a philosophical difference.

One style of EAP, primarily associated with practitioners trained in the Equine Assisted Growth and Learning Association (EAGALA) model, involves a licensed mental health practitioner working alongside an equine specialist. EAGALA sessions follow a structured plan incorporating group challenges and tasks. In the EAGALA model, all activities with the horses are conducted on the ground and there is no mounted work. Although EAGALA are not the only organization to offer this type of training, they are perhaps the most widely known. The focus in this approach is on the problem solving and experiential process rather than on the horse–human relationship. The aim is to highlight the roles and responsibilities that people take within groups as a metaphor for what they might experience outside of therapy. In this model, the role of the mental health practitioner within the EAP setting is to hold the space for the process to unfold, provide instructions for the activity, and highlight these metaphors, whilst observing, and interpreting the participant's actions at the end of the activity. The role of the equine specialist within the EAP setting is to focus on the horses' behaviors and the physical safety of the participants. It is important to note that there are also other models of EAP that offer more focus on a relational and experiential approach, without a defined equine specialist role, and with mounted work included as well as work on the ground.

In contrast, EFP incorporates a broad range of therapeutic approaches and experiential elements to the process, and provides a much less rigid structure of session planning and designs than EAP. EFP highlights the relational aspects of the horse–human encounter and views the horse as a cofacilitator in the therapeutic process, emphasizing the innate wisdom of the horse and the power of a living being bearing witness. Leigh Shambo, author of *The Listening Heart*, positioned the process in this way:

> *The practitioner, trained to recognize developmental and psychological issues of particular individuals, will work within the core affective dimensions most relevant to the client, and view the horse as a flexible, always respected partner in healing.*

EFP, in general, is a more embodied approach with practitioners focusing on not just the nonverbal communication with the horses, but also the nonverbal, body awareness, and sensations for the client. These embodied encounters within the EFP session range from simply standing in the presence of the horse(s), grooming and feeding, mucking out stalls, or sitting bareback on a horse, to conducting exercises with the horse whilst on the ground, or riding the horse. EFP sessions may include both a licensed mental health professional and an equine specialist, but the therapist can also be dually credentialed as the equine professional. EFP may be conducted with individuals, couples, families, or groups for a wide range of populations.

Theoretical perspectives and client populations

A review of the literature indicates that EAP and EFP practitioners stem from a wide range of theoretical perspectives, serving a diverse range of clients. Kay Trotter's book, *Harnessing the Power of Equine Assisted Counseling*, is a collection of case studies, research, and clinical techniques by EFMHS practitioners, and at a glance does not reveal any particular pattern of matching theoretical perspectives to EAP/EFP approach. Contributors include clinical psychologists, licensed professional counselors, licensed social workers, licensed marriage and family therapists, psychoanalysts, substance abuse counselors, play therapists, and somatic practitioners. Populations served include trauma, attachment, sexual abuse, children and adolescents, addiction, anxiety, depression, and ADHD. Many of these practitioners developed their own certification programs, methods, and techniques within the general frameworks of EAP or EFP. This highlights the need for more research, both in terms of assessing efficacy and in finding a way to unite the increasingly fragmented field of EFMHS.

THE HERD INSTITUTE MODEL OF EFP

At the HERD Institute, we believe that the role of the EFP practitioner is to facilitate a relationship between the horse and the client, and reflect back to the client what the practitioner is witnessing during this process to support the client's therapeutic journey. The HERD Institute Model is an embodied approach where practitioners are focusing on not just the nonverbal communication with the horses, but also the nonverbal, body awareness, and sensations for the client. In contrast to EAP where the activities for the session are usually planned in advance, the experiential elements during an EFP session often arise in the moment, as a collaborative experiment between the client, horse, and practitioner. At the center of the HERD Institute Model are the philosophical foundations of an embodied, relational, and authentic way of being.

Chapter 3

Philosophical Foundations

The only thing we require to be good philosophers is the faculty of wonder... Most adults accept the world as a matter of course. This is precisely where philosophers are a notable exception. A philosopher never gets quite used to the world. To him or her, the world continues to seem a bit unreasonable - bewildering, even enigmatic. Philosophers and small children thus have an important faculty in common.

(Jostein Gaarder, Sophie's World)

Equine Facilitated Psychotherapy and Learning (EFPL) is currently an umbrella term for the eclectic mix of various disciplines and theories that incorporate horses into clinical, educational, and organizational work with a diverse range of clients. Students and practitioners of EFPL come from all walks of life and are licensed psychologists, social workers, counselors, educators, coaches, and corporate trainers, all working from a different philosophical and theoretical origin, with the common belief that the interaction with horses brings healing, learning, and personal development for clients. They may or may not work in partnership with an equine specialist, whose role varies from solely providing safety for equines and humans during sessions, to being a fully integrated part of the facilitation process. The equine specialist is often not a trained facilitator or mental health practitioner. The mental health practitioner, educator, or trainer, may not be an experienced horse person. This not only brings a wealth of knowledge and skills into the modality, but also offers up challenges in terms of epistemology, ontology, and ethics. How do we know if what we do is consistent with our philosophical foundations? Does our way of working represent a coherent framework that reflects our values and beliefs, or is it a mix of ideas gleaned from different, and possibly contradicting, philosophies?

This chapter aims to critically assess these gaps and inconsistencies, and outline the philosophical foundations of the HERD approach to EFPL.

PHILOSOPHICAL RELEVANCE

What is the relevance of a chapter on philosophy in a book on EFPL? Philosophy is often seen as an obscure and exclusionary language, limited to the realms of the ivory towers of academia, and much too abstract for the

Equine-Facilitated Psychotherapy and Learning. DOI: http://dx.doi.org/10.1016/B978-0-12-812601-1.00003-1

application of everyday life. It is a complex discipline that examines the mysteries of existence and reality, and explores the relationships between humanity and nature, and self and environment. In this chapter, I want to shift the paradigm so that philosophy is acknowledged for what it is: the central foundations for all that we believe, cultivated from an attitude of awe and wonder for the world we live in. Philosophy challenges us to think deeply, more critically, and to live with integrity. It is, in fact, the perfect starting point for all our interactions with horses, so that we can stand clear in what we believe in as a modality.

As EFPL practitioners, we are most concerned with how to bring what we know about horses and human relationships into a meaningful experience with our clients, to support therapeutic growth or learning, whilst adhering to our ethical principles. Philosophy examines what we know (ontology), and how we know what we know (epistemology). It also challenges us to consider what we should do with what we know (ethics), and how we experience it (phenomenology). Examining our philosophical assumptions allows us to offer empirical evidence that is much needed within the field of EFPL, and helps us to translate this into practice.

Existing literature on EFPL has integrated philosophical language into its vocabulary, often through a process of appropriation and introjection without much discourse. We refer to horses as authentic beings who mirror our emotions through being embodied in their relationships, and describe the I-Thou encounters with these majestic partners with the assumption that we are all speaking from the same page. These are philosophical terms with specific meanings that have a direct impact on how we work with our clients and horses, so it is imperative that we understand them. In reality, there may be fundamental differences in our personal philosophies from which we approach the work that may appear as outward inconsistencies, and may reduce the validity of our modality in the eyes of our mental health and other professional colleagues who work outside of the equine facilitated domain. It is time to unpack these assumptions and examine how they fit with our underlying beliefs.

Human Animals

Firstly, we need to address the language we use that defines our relationship with other living beings. Regarding the interactions with and interconnection of humans and animals, anthropologist Barbara King comments that:

> Of course, we humans *are* animals... The mutual relating we engage in with other animals transforms us, yes, but that transformation rests squarely in the common trajectory that we share with other creatures. We, all of us, have evolved, and changed over time. *Homo sapiens*...evolved to think and feel with *other* animals right from the start. To explore being with animals is to explore our own past.

Philosophers throughout the ages have offered countless musings about what it means to be human, and what separates us, human beings, from all the other creatures with whom we share this Earth. Whether it is our ability to understand language, good versus evil, love, or death, Mark Rowland, a modern philosopher, suggested that these are all simply stories that we tell; that the actual difference between humans and other animals is that "humans are the animals that believe the stories they tell themselves." While this discussion does not focus on what it means to be human, it is important to acknowledge the human animal as a species that shares space with so many others. With this clarification in mind, we can refer to human animals as humans, and non-human animals as animals, and explore the philosophical foundations of the experience of being humans who have relationships with animals. In this way, we can be respectful of the "who" of the animal rather than objectifying them in a way that precludes any relationship or notion that they are sentient beings with their own feelings. Carl Safina, a world-renowned ecologist says that it has become so popular to separate out "human" emotions when talking about animals that we have forgotten that human emotions *are* animal emotions, made of the same sensations and inherited nervous systems through our evolution. This is not to say that it is accurate to ascribe human emotions onto other animal species, but to acknowledge our shared evolutionary trajectory as well as our species-specific traits and attributes. For this, we turn to a philosophical tradition called phenomenology.

PHENOMENOLOGY AND EMBODIMENT

Phenomenology, a branch of philosophy pertaining to the study *of* experience and *how* we experience was developed in the 20th century by Edmund Husserl, a German philosopher, who was interested in the structures of consciousness. Husserl focused on the idea that all experience is subjective (from an individual's own perspective). Taken from the Greek word "phainomenon," meaning "appearances," phenomenology can be understood as the study of the perception of experience. This includes both passive experiences such as sensations, as well as more active processes such as imagination, behaviors, emotions, and thoughts that lead to the concept of intentionality (the belief that all experience is directed toward something/someone external to ourselves). In other words, phenomenology is the study of consciousness *as it is lived through and experienced in awareness.*

Maurice Merleau-Ponty is often credited in modern European philosophy for bringing the body into focus through his rejection of the Cartesian split between mind and body, and the introduction of phenomenology as an embodied experience. His magnum opus, *Phenomenology of Perception*, was built upon Husserl's concept of phenomenology through incorporating the concept of an intersubjective, bodily experience that is situated in time and space. He said that:

> We have relearned to feel our body; we have found underneath the objective and detached knowledge of the body that other knowledge which we have of it in virtue of its always being with us and of the fact that *we are our body*. In the same way we shall need to reawaken our experience of the world as it appears to us in so far as we are in the world through our body, and in so far as we perceive the world *with* our body. But by thus remaking contact with the body and with the world, we shall also rediscover ourself, since, perceiving as we do with our body, the body is a natural self and, as it were, the subject of perception.

In this, Merleau-Ponty was way ahead of his time as current research and neuroscience is now able to support this theory that challenges Descarte's assertion that "I think, therefore, I am," and provides evidence that consciousness is experienced through our body as a holistic event rather than a mental representation of the external environment, and that the mind is inextricably part of the body. Merleau-Ponty argued that our body *is* our perception and way of being, pointing to the paradoxical nature of perception always being from within a particular perspective. In this way, we can begin to acknowledge that our experiencing of ourselves, even on a descriptive level, is the experiencing of our consciousness. This idea has a direct impact on clinical applications and challenges our ideas of what we mean when we refer to "the self" and "relationship." We will discuss this in more detail in the next chapter.

So the living body acts as a mediator between our own perspective and the world, where the body is the experience of our self that connects with the world through intentionality. It is the body that provides the intentional threads that connect us to our surroundings, revealing to us that we are the perceiver and the perceived. Perception is based in behavior by way of being a sentient body that acts with intentionality with the world around it. In other words, it is always already situated within and with the environment, and is an active agent in that environment. Intentionality, in this sense, is the bodily orientation, direction, and/or movement towards something in the environment.

Phenomenologically speaking, embodiment cannot be a static process as the body is experienced spatially and temporally. As Merleau-Ponty points out:

> How the body inhabits space (and time, for that matter) can be seen more clearly by considering the body in motion because movement is not content with passively undergoing space and time, it actively assumes them, it takes them up in their original signification that is effaced in the banality of established situations.

As such, movement and perception are interdependent, one upon the other, as a phenomenon of the body. A phenomenology of perception is, therefore, an embodied perception, and is a descriptive account of the experience *as it is* without reference to psychological origins and causal assumptions of preexisting structures and theories. This translates into clinical practice as a non-interpretative process that focuses on the description of the experience.

EFPL and Phenomenology

The HERD approach to EFPL takes this philosophy of phenomenological attitude as a framework for the equine-facilitated encounter. Drawing from Gestalt psychotherapy theory, the application of a phenomenological attitude to the therapeutic and/or learning process is one that acknowledges that clients bring with them their own subjective experiences. Rather than interpreting what is happening for them, the aim is to facilitate an increase in their own awareness of how they make meaning of their experiences for themselves. We will discuss this in more detail in the next chapter.

Phenomenology of Animal of Life

In bringing together the philosophical and theoretical strands, it is necessary to include a discussion on the phenomenology of animal life. Since the HERD Model approaches the process phenomenologically by viewing the client's experiences as unique to him/her, we must also consider the experience of the horse(s) in the interaction. In other words, a consideration of what the horse(s) are experiencing becomes part of what holds our curiosity during the process. This occurs not only as theoretical application, but stems from the philosophical stance that Merleau-Ponty drew from Uexküll's *Umwelt* theory (where organisms are deemed to experience living in their own species-specific ways of being-in-the-world) that "the being of the animal lodges itself in the development of their ontologies." Merleau-Ponty referred to the common ground between human and animal lives as a strange kinship that emphasizes the bidirectional nature of the relationship:

> *Animals inhabit our surrounding world in which their lived bodies and lively subjectivities are manifest. Indeed, they cannot be fully understood when only examined in their objective physical or behavioural characteristics; a transcendental method is needed.*

Umwelt, in this sense, is seen as the self-organizing principle that explains both the animal's physicality and behavior (i.e., what makes a horse a horse), such that the relationship between the animal and its surroundings becomes one of meaning. This strange kinship leads to an intersubjective and collective endeavor whose meaningfulness is shared "not only among humans possessing language, but among numerous intentional, responsive, interpreting animals with whom we share our lives."

EFPL and Phenomenology of Animal Life

The challenge that occurs when applying this philosophical lens to practical application within EFPL is in the attempt to draw meanings from the horse's behavior during the encounter. Whilst the client holds their phenomenal experience (i.e., their individual perspective) and can make meaning for him/herself, and part of the task for the practitioner is to raise the client's awareness of this, the horse's phenomenal experience is essentially still one of relative mystery. For this conundrum, we turn to Scott Churchill's theory of *second-person perspectivity* and its relation to embodiment. Firmly situated within the phenomenological paradigm, Churchill suggested that a second-person perspective allows one to resonate with the experience of the other through an embodied encounter as a way of phenomenological inquiry, whether this other is human or animal. By stepping outside of one's own perspective and focusing on the other's intentional communicative gestures and behaviors, the encounter is deepened. Speaking of his experiences of working with Bonobos, Churchill believes that our experience with animals can be transformed:

> *when we step up real close, closer than others do, putting our faces and our bodies right up to the glass, standing on the animal's level..."touching" each other while looking into each other's eyes. There is a feeling of mutual respect that humbles one in such moments. A sense of fidelity to the animal other's nature as soul-brother calls one to consider one's own ethics in one's dealing with all animals.*

The HERD approach to EFPL adheres to this phenomenological philosophy as a mode of inquiry into the therapeutic and learning encounters, not only for the client but also for the horse(s) involved. This embodied exploration of being with another being in each moment provides the starting point for healing and growth.

BUBER'S *I-THOU*

Martin Buber was a religious existentialist who expressed his philosophy as a synthesis of Hasidic Judaism and existentialism, where his utmost concern was the difference between mere existence and authentic existence. Transposing his notions of receptivity and dialogue towards God into a way of approaching fellow human beings, Buber, in his seminal work *I and Thou*, elucidated his philosophy of dialogue as the ontological foundation of existence. He distinguished between two primary relationships of *I-Thou* and *I-It*, which he called "primary words," and suggested that these are the relational attitudes from which human beings interact with the world. The *I-Thou* stance refers to a meeting in which one approaches the other as another being (a "who"), and the *I-It* refers to the turning of the other into an object, or de-humanized and inanimate "thing." Dialogue, in this context, is not only the spoken word but refers to all interactions between self and other as one exists in the world; it is in our way of being and experiencing:

> Through the meeting that which confronts me is fulfilled, and encounters the world of things, there to be endlessly active, endlessly to become *It,* but also endlessly to become *Thou* again, inspiring and blessing. It is "embodied"; its body emerges from the flow of the spaceless, timeless present on the shore of existence.

Much like Merleau-Ponty's embodied phenomenology, this is a holistic engagement with the world within which we are always already situated and to which we are always belonging. The *I-Thou* stance necessitates a shared perspective; rather than looking *at* the other, it is looking *with*.

From Buber's perspective, not only does life occur in the space between self and other, but more importantly it acts as the catalyst of the *formation* of both self and other, and whatever emerges in the *between* is where the meaning of inter-relatedness is found. In this way, authentic existence is not something that occurs for the individual, nor is it a social concept; rather, it is a function of the process of relationships happening in the between:

> Primary words do not signify things, but they intimate relations. Primary words do not describe something that might exist independently of them, but being spoken they bring about existence. Primary words are spoken from the being. If *Thou* is said, the *I* of the *I-Thou* is said along with it. If *It* is said, the *I* of the *I-It* is said along with it. The primary word *I-Thou* can only be said with the whole being. The primary word *I-It* can never be spoken with the whole being.

For Buber, authentic existence is only possible within the *I-Thou* relationship. This requires both beings to bring themselves wholly into the moment of meeting. It is this embodied mutuality of connection that allows for the authentic existence of both beings to emerge. The *I-It* relationship is not an authentic existence by its nature of approaching the other as a separate entity and without mutuality in relationship to the *I*. While authentic existence emerges within the *I-Thou,* Buber acknowledged that that way of being is neither a sustainable one, nor is it one for which one can strive:

> The *Thou* meets me through grace – it is not found by seeking...but I step into direct relation with it. Hence the relation means being chosen and choosing ... I become through my relation to the *Thou;* as I become *I,* I say *Thou.* All real living is meeting.

These *I-Thou* meetings are grounded in the present moment and can only be experienced in the here-and-now with the whole of our being. In this way, existence becomes the fluid movement between the *I-Thou* and *I-It* moments in life, while acknowledging the impermanence of those authentic moments. An *I*-Thou moment may also evaporate into an *I-It* when one becomes absorbed within oneself through what Buber called *reflexion*, where the experience of the other becomes focused only on one's own experience, such that one allows the other to exist only as part of oneself. Thus, all who are *Thou* after the relational moment becomes an *It*, and any *It* stepping into relationship becomes a *Thou*. As such, Buber's perspective regarding engagement with the world can be seen as an embodied authenticity of each moment, as "He who gives himself to it may withhold nothing of himself." In this way authentic dialogue is an embodied and intentional act "where each of the participants really has in mind the other or others in their present and particular being and turns to them with the intention of establishing a living mutual relation between himself and them," that may manifest through not only words, but silence too, and leads to the embodiment of authentic living. For Buber, being embodied in this way is to be present with the other in the fullness of existence. To embody this authentic presence is to commit to an attitude of inclusion such that:

> Not only is the shared silence of two such persons a dialogue, but also their dialogical life continues, even when they are separated in space, as the continual potential presence of the one to the other, as an unexpressed intercourse.

From Buber's perspective, the search for an embodied authenticity is both an ontological and phenomenal activity that acknowledges the spatiality and temporality of each moment; the process of always already being a relational body-in-the-world can only lead to a fleeting quality of embodied authentic existence:

> This presence before which I am placed changes its form, its appearance, its revelation, they are different from myself...If I stand up to them, concern myself with them, meet them in a real way, that is, with the truth of my whole life, then and only then am I "really" there: I am there if I am there, and where this "there" is, is always determined less by myself than by the presence of this being which changes its form and its appearance.

Authenticity, in this context, is taken to be the process through which one steps into that fleeting quality of authentic existence in the way that Buber described, and as an embodied authentic process. Thus, to embody authenticity includes the risk that one takes in choosing to step into relationships knowing that it will bring about change in oneself. This unity of experiencing complements the intersubjectivity of Merleau-Ponty's embodied phenomenology and emphasizes:

> He who takes his stand in relation shares in a reality, that is, in a being that neither merely belongs to him nor merely lies outside him. All reality is an activity in which I share without being able to appropriate for myself. Where there is no sharing, there is no reality. Where there is self-appropriation there is no reality. The more direct the contact with the *Thou*, the fuller is the sharing.

Embodying that reality is acknowledging that the body is an intentional body, instinctively relational, and cocreated with the other in the relationship as inherently full of implicit meanings and relational understandings.

Embodied Connections of Phenomenology and *I-Thou*

Of the commonalities between phenomenology and *I-Thou*, the languaging of the embodied experience is the biggest challenge. This difficulty in giving language to the bodily experience as a nature of embodiment also extends to the holistic and intersubjective dimension within the two philosophies, all of which combine to provide a framework for the theoretical principles within the HERD approach. In transposing the philosophy of embodied authenticity into the theory and practice of EFPL, it highlights the importance of how practitioners bring themselves into these encounters in an embodied and authentic manner. Foundational to this approach is the inescapable relational aspect of living in an always already situated time-and-space that cocreates, not only our way of being in the world and the world itself, but also our way of experiencing the world, as living, breathing, and sentient beings.

BUBER'S *I-THOU* AND HORSES

Significant for the HERD approach to EFPL, Buber's conceptualization of the *I-Thou* encounter emerged from his own interactions with a horse. As a young boy, Buber visited his grandparent's farm where he experienced stroking a horse to whom he was particularly drawn:

> I must say that what I experienced in touch with the animal was the Other...When I stroked the mighty mane, sometimes, marvelously smooth-combed, at other times just as astonishingly wild, and felt the life beneath my hand it was as though the element of vitality itself bordered on my skin, something that was not I, was certainly not akin to me, palpably the other, not just another, really the Other itself; and yet it let me approach, confided itself to me, placed itself elementally in the relation of *Thou* and *Thou* with me.

As he continued stroking the horse, he began to notice the difference in quality of connection with the horse when he allowed himself to be fully present with the horse, and how the horse also disconnected from him when his mind drifted to other things. "But once...it struck me about the stroking, what fun it gave me, and suddenly I became conscious of my hand. The game went on as before, but something had changed, it was no longer the same thing."

Discovery of *I-It* Encounters

This experience prompted his formulation of the difference between an *I-Thou* and *I-It* encounter, and is significant for the HERD approach in bringing the philosophical tenants of the *I-Thou* relationship into the work with clients and horses. This is not based on an anthropocentric belief, and in fact, is quite the opposite; to step into an *I-Thou* relation with a non human animal is to acknowledge that humans are not the measure of all things. With the growing evidence on the therapeutic benefits of human-animal bonds and the physiological impact of being with horses, it is possible to view the connections made between clients and horses through an *I-Thou* lens. As with human-to-human relationships, there is a continuous flow between the *I-Thou* and *I-It*, during an EFPL session. The HERD approach focuses on increasing awareness of these shifts in each moment as a way to enable clients to embody their ability to connect and disconnect in their relationships.

Chapter 4

Theoretical Foundations

BROADENING HORIZONS AND DIGGING DEEP

My first experience to the world of equine assisted psychotherapy was a 1-day introduction session in the United Kingdom, led by an EAGALA therapist and equine specialist. Working with two horses in an indoor arena, the group was set a specific task and took turns to navigate the challenge in silence before talking about what had happened for each participant individually. Whilst I enjoyed the experience, I was left with a yearning for a more relational way of working, and missed the immediacy of attending to the here-and-now process between group members in the way that I was familiar with in a Gestalt therapy setting. So I began my wider search for something that fitted my personal and professional philosophy, and found the Gestalt Equine Institute of the Rockies. Their 2-year certification program equipped me to integrate my already in-depth Gestalt training into incorporating this way of working with horses. In my quest to immerse myself deeper into this field, I completed my PhD in Psychology with a specialization in Existential, Humanistic, and Transpersonal Psychology (researching the embodied experiences of Equine-Facilitated Psychotherapy), enrolled in an intensive mentorship program with Barbara Rector, became a PATH International Registered Therapeutic Riding Instructor, and engaged with the corporate equine assisted learning environment through the European Association for Horse Assisted Education community. All of these experiences have contributed to both broadening my horizons, and simultaneously, deepening my philosophical and theoretical understanding of this work. The Human-Equine Relational Development (HERD) approach to Equine-Facilitated Psychotherapy and Learning (EFPL) is the result of a truly integrative, holistic, relational, and embodied approach that is underpinned by a cohesive philosophy that translates into applicable theory and empirical research. This chapter discusses the core theory behind the HERD approach to EFPL, and how the philosophical concepts of phenomenology and I-Thou are integral to these theoretical foundations.

CORE THEORY

There are three central tenets within the HERD approach to EFPL that are based on Existential-Humanistic Psychology and Gestalt Psychotherapy

Equine-Facilitated Psychotherapy and Learning. DOI: http://dx.doi.org/10.1016/B978-0-12-812601-1.00004-3

principles. I like to refer to them as: The Here & Now; What & How; and I-Thou. Together, these three pillars offer a framework for practice that promotes an increase in embodied awareness, which in turn leads to the ability to form and sustain deeper, more connected, and meaningful relationships. Whilst these are psychological theories that have emerged within the context of therapy, they are also equally relevant within the context of organizational training and educational environments.

Here and Now

Fritz Perls, most often credited as the founder of Gestalt therapy believed that "What is essential is not that the therapist learn something about the patient and then teach it to him, but that the therapist teach the patient *how* to learn about himself." The existential focus is on how a client is negotiating their experience of being alive in full awareness of the moment; it is paying attention to the process of the session in each moment as it unfolds, rather than on the content that the client offers; and the experience of the past as it emerges in the present moment, rather than talking about past events in the there-and-then. Existential therapist, Irv Yalom, distinguished between the two phases of working in the here-and-now as: *actively calling attention* to the present moment, and the *illumination of the process* in the moment. This lived experience offers clients new awareness of how they are responding to their life situations and their sense of self.

Within a therapeutic encounter, rather than asking clients to tell their stories in a way that takes them into their histories, and instead paying attention to the process in the moment provides the practitioner with valuable information. Since whatever is being experienced in the moment is what is readily available to be drawn attention to, the process of the encounter is the key to unlocking the clients' awareness of the choices they are making in their lives. According to Laura Perls, one of the cofounders of Gestalt therapy, this way of working "deals with the obvious, with what is *immediately* available to the awareness of client or therapist and can be shared and expanded in the actual ongoing communication."

Awareness

Within the HERD approach to EFPL, there is an emphasis on increasing awareness of the here-and-now in any given situation. But what does that actually mean? According to Gestalt therapist, Gary Yontef, awareness can be seen as the way an individual experiences and interprets the here and now; their understanding of what they are doing, and how they are doing it. Furthermore, it is their knowledge that they are responsible for their actions and their choice of action. In other words, it is a deliberate and conscious act of paying attention to physical sensations, feelings, and imaginations about what is happening to me, and the environment I am integrated in.

For a deeper exploration of this, we turn to the integration of the philosophical concept of phenomenology into psychological theory.

What and How

As discussed in the previous chapter, Merleau-Ponty developed the phenomenological method to include descriptions arising from the body, including physical sensations as expressions. Integrating this concept into psychological theory allows for the practitioner to work from an embodied perspective so that the therapeutic relationship becomes a whole-bodied encounter.

This phenomenological approach is fundamental to the HERD approach to EFPL, where the therapeutic stance is to remain descriptive, not speculative, or interpretive. This process of attending to what *is* allows the therapist to enter into the world of the client and experience the world through them. Coupled with attending to what is happening in the here and now, and staying with the process as it unfolds, the therapist can facilitate a deeper level of understanding for the client. Since we all make meaning of our experiences from our own individual perspectives (i.e., our phenomenal experience), past experiences will affect the way an individual acts and reacts to stimuli in the here and now.

The HERD approach promotes the theory that first there is awareness, and then there is choice. The practitioner draws the client's attention to what is happening in the moment, both internally (sensations and emotions) and relationally (with others), focusing on the quality of connection between the client and their environment. In this way, we can focus our attention on **what** is happening for the client and **how** it impacts him or her. This phenomenological approach requires the practitioner to take a holistic stance to become fully immersed in the experience of the client.

Holism

The HERD approach to EFPL subscribes to the notion that human beings experience the world by interpreting, or drawing meaning from, what is around them and *even if the picture is incomplete*, an individual's natural tendency will be to attempt to complete it. This is exemplified in the idea that the whole is greater than the sum of its parts. Fritz Perls, convinced that examining isolated parts of the client was not adequate in the search of understanding the essence of the whole person, formulated the concept of figure/ground: The figure is what is present in our awareness in any particular moment, and the (back)ground is the context of our experiences from which we draw meaning. This is a dynamic process as the same background can give rise to different figures of interest. Imagine a lava lamp as it flows and forms different shapes within its structure on a continuous basis.

This concept of figure/ground is indicative of Merleau-Ponty's influence on Gestalt theory as it emphasizes the already situated aspect of embodied living that is experienced as shifts in awareness from one figure to another. The dance between figure/background provides the practitioner with information on what is happening for the client and how it is impacting them. So our attention is constantly shifting from the background to what becomes figural in the moment. It is in the identification of the figure and the associated ground that any fixed patterns of behavior (or fixed gestalts) reveal themselves, and any unfinished business can be completed and experienced in awareness in the here and now.

Through the use of three main techniques, the therapist aims to uncover the client's personal experience of the world in each particular situation (figure) *for them* (against their background), thus increasing their awareness and personal growth. The three aspects of the phenomenological approach are bracketing, description, and horizontalism.

Bracketing (also referred to as epoché) is the process whereby the therapist attempts as much as possible to clear their mind of any distractions from the here and now with the client, and is a vital skill practiced within the HERD approach to EFPL. By putting aside notions of therapist-as-expert, and any distractions, assumptions, or judgments we may have of what the client is saying or doing, we can be more present in the moment with them.

At first glance, this idea may seem contradictory to the notion of phenomenology. If as human beings we naturally make meanings from situations, and perceive things as they are for ourselves, then how can we as therapists stop that process? The idea of bracketing however, is not to ignore this trait in human beings to make meaning, but merely to be aware of any preconceptions which may surface in our minds, and to consciously put them to one side as we work with our client, thereby allowing ourselves to be more present and available to the client in the here and now, and to ascertain what meaning is being made by the client and how he/she is responding to the situation in that moment.

The second technique in the phenomenological approach is that of description. Again, based on the theory that individuals naturally make meaning from a given situation, it is a necessary skill for a therapist to be able to describe a situation without judgment or interpretation, in order for them to be open to the lived experience of the client. More importantly, when the therapist purely describes a situation and avoids putting any interpretation on things, it allows *the client* to explore their own phenomenal experience. As that happens in the here and now, the client may then be able to observe their own reactions, or fixed patterns of behavior, and the therapist can support the client to explore this. In this way, clients are encouraged to find their own agency and become more conscious of the choices they are making in their lives.

The third aspect of the phenomenological approach is that of horizontalism or equalization. This means that every observation by the therapist is given the same importance and works in a similar way to bracketing, in that the therapist must suspend judgment on what to assign priority. This technique allows the therapist to look at the whole picture given to them in the form of the client. This means paying attention to everything, the figure, and the ground, and to what is missing as well as to what is present. This intricate dance between therapist and client allows for authenticity to emerge in what Yalom refers to as "the between," and supports the development of a deeper connection within the relationship. It is also in "the between" that the therapist can hold an I-Thou attitude towards the client.

I-Thou

As discussed in the previous chapter, Martin Buber's philosophy of I-Thou plays an important role in the emergence of authenticity. Applying this philosophy within the context of psychological theory requires that the practitioner meet the client as a fellow traveler on a shared journey. Rather than stepping into the "role" of therapist, this model requires the therapist to bring him/herself authentically into the encounter on an embodied level. James Bugental, one of the founders of the existential-humanistic psychology approach, believed that by accessing one's subjectivity more fully, individuals could reclaim contact with their inner experiencing, which has the potential to guide them towards authentic living. Kierkegaard and Sartre spoke of authenticity as being in touch with one's self and of having the conviction and passion to choose to live an authentic life while resisting the leveling effect of mass-culture. These perspectives of authenticity have at their core an assumption generally shared within existential-humanistic therapy of the concept of self as a continuous process and not a fixed entity.

The HERD approach is founded on the principles of the relational encounter and emphasizes the importance of the therapist's presence. By integrating Buber's I-Thou philosophy, the authentic presence of the therapist invokes and motivates the client to become present in the encounter, leading to a new awakened experience of living for them in that moment. An embodied way-of-being allows for authentic living that incorporates true connection and contact with another being. Contact, in this context, is the process of making connection with another in the quality of meeting proposed by Buber's *I-Thou* moment. Gestalt therapists, Polster and Polster, captured the essence of this in their description of contact as "not just togetherness or joining. It can only happen between separate beings, always requiring independence and always risking the capture of union...I am no longer only me, but me and thee make we." It is in taking this risk, and engaging with what emerges in the between, where the meaning of the interhuman phenomena can be found. Peter Philippson, a leading Gestalt therapist in the United Kingdom, refers to this wholly embodied process as self in relation.

Lost in Translation

In our quest to honor our intentions of adhering to our philosophical beliefs, there is often a paradoxical disconnect between philosophical foundations, theory, and practice. It is important to understand that within the philosophical traditions of embodied phenomenology and Buber's *I-Thou* attitude to relating, that practitioners do not translate this process to idealize an embodied, authentic, *I-Thou* connection. What I mean by this is that it would be easy for students of this approach to turn the *I-Thou* connection into an aim for the client. Paradoxically, not only does this remove the possibility for such a connection, as the process becomes one of achieving an agenda rather than honoring the client's process, but in fact becomes a distortion of Buber's philosophy which emphasizes the importance of the movement between the *I-Thou* and *I-It* ways of relating, and acknowledges the impermanence of the *I-Thou* moment. In the attempt to hold on to that moment, we have already moved into an *I-It*.

The HERD approach brings into focus the movement between these moments, paying attention to the embodied nature of the encounters for both the clients and the horses. By honoring the philosophical framework that supports this process, we can translate this into theoretical concepts that reflect our beliefs, and in turn, apply them in praxis.

EMBODIMENT AND AUTHENTICITY

There is much debate within existential-humanistic psychology as to what authenticity is and how one can live an authentic life. Definitions of authenticity relate to the fundamental questions of self-concept and the idea of a true self. However, in the quest to find one's true self, one may be hampered by other's expectations and desires that are incongruent with one's own. At the same time, if self-actualization is the path to authentic living, then succumbing to external influences is seen as the road to an inauthentic life.

James Bugental suggests that,

Authenticity does not consist of rejection of the familiar world. It does not call for one to deny values, activities, associates, or any aspect of his/her life, but through active participation. This allows for what Kirk Schneider, a leading existential-humanistic psychologist, calls an "experiential liberation" that encompasses a holistic engagement of being in the present moment. It is a full-bodied process where "clients are supported to "reoccupy" (i.e., embody) the parts of themselves that have been denied. The more that clients are able to reoccupy themselves, the more they are able to both access and express hitherto estranged dimensions of themselves, and it is these very dimensions that deepen people's appreciation for life."

This experiential liberation challenges the Cartesian duality of a mind-body split and the reliance on cognitive, rational, and logical interpretation of the lived experience, and unifies the experience of being-in-the-world in an embodied way. This unified experience naturally incorporates both the intrapersonal and the interpersonal domain.

THE EMBODIED RELATIONAL SELF

Fully connecting with another involves being in the encounter in a fully embodied way such that it takes into account the physical, emotional, and cognitive sense of oneself in relation to another in each moment. It includes: (a) *interoception*, which involves the visceral body response to the outer world, (b) *proprioception*, which relates to the body's balance and equilibrium, along with a sense of how the parts of the body are experienced in relation to other parts of the body, and (c) *movement*, which informs the person of the body's motion in relation to surroundings.

Gestalt psychotherapist, James Kepner, offered an experiential and phenomenological view of body psychotherapy that echoes Merleau-Ponty's embodied phenomenology, where:

> *Experience of our body is experience of our self, just as our thinking, imagery, and ideas are part of our self...When we make our body experience an "it" instead of "I", we make ourselves less than we are. We become diminished...our bodily being is intrinsic to our relationship to our world.*

The Gestalt use of the term "embodied" takes into account the fullness of one's experience of one self, internally and externally, in relation to their environment and acknowledges that I *am* my body and that my body *is* me. This means that as one's body moves and transforms, so does one's self, so that the internal experiencing of one's self and one's relationship to everyone and the environment is altered. This is referred to as our **felt sense**, and highlights the embodiment of our lived experience and the process by which we do that *and* points to a more intuitive and implicit knowledge of ourselves. Thus, the continuous nature of the self as process incorporates the bodily experience as well as information from our environment that is yet to be processed. Peter Levine, founder of the Somatic Experiencing method, proposes that living in an embodied way can be seen as

> *gaining, through the vehicle of awareness, the capacity to feel the ambient physical sensations of unfettered energy and aliveness as they pulse through our bodies. It is here that mind and body, thought and feeling, psyche and spirit, are held together, welded in an undifferentiated unity of experience*

The HERD approach to EFPL emphasizes the increased awareness of **self, other, and environment.** The task of the practitioner is in supporting clients to rediscover the fullness and authenticity of their selves through this embodied awareness.

Chapter 5

Theoretical Foundations II: Where Does the Horse Fit in?

THE MAGIC OF HORSES

There are many believers within the field of Equine-Facilitated Psychotherapy and Learning (EFPL) who subscribe to the idea that horses embody a higher wisdom, that they are spiritual beings that act as a medium to the Universe for us lesser human beings. Many others believe that horses are the mirrors to our souls, capable of seeing past any façade we may present to the world, reaching into our hidden vulnerabilities to illuminate our deepest desires. Most of us have come into the field through a deep love and respect for horses, with personal experiences and relationships with these incredible animals that have altered us at our core, and the belief that their authentic way of being-in-the-world can support us to find deeper meaning in our lives. There are so many stories I could tell about the wisdom and synchronicity I have witnessed with clients when interacting with horses. Several of my clients refer to the process as "Horse Magic." I have heard many more accounts of seemingly improbable actions by these awe-inspiring animals that confirm for me that with horses, there is more than meets the eye. Yet there are others who maintain a safe distance from the more spiritual and "alternative" explanations of how and why horses are able to bring about such deep transformations, preferring instead to focus on finding evidence-based and scientific proof. Personally, while I acknowledge that our field is lacking in the types of scientific inquiry that brings us credibility to those outside of the EFPL environment, I also believe that the qualitative, felt sense, and embodied experience provides a much more compelling description, transforming that which is so intangible to something profoundly meaningful. One of my most astounding experiences occurred several years ago, and captures the essence of the philosophy and theory at the heart of this book.

Not long after moving to the States, I attended a training session at the Gestalt Equine Institute of the Rockies. The institute had recently moved locations and we were about to go out to the corrals to meet the herd for the first time. I was desperately grieving the loss of my pony, Rupert, after leaving him behind in the United Kingdom when we moved to the States. I was adamant that I was not ready to open my heart to another horse,

Equine-Facilitated Psychotherapy and Learning. DOI: http://dx.doi.org/10.1016/B978-0-12-812601-1.00005-5

and had explicitly given myself time to grieve fully and openly. Although Rupert did not belong to me, I had leased him for a couple of years, and leaving him was by far the hardest aspect of our international relocation. Family and friends understood where we were, and with the convenience of technology, they were able to keep in contact through email, social media, and the telephone. As far as Rupert was concerned, I was convinced that his experience was one of abandonment. Where once I would see him every day, suddenly I disappeared. My only consolation was that his owner had promised that I could go and visit him whenever I traveled back home to the United Kingdom. So I was heartbroken when I heard through the grapevine, the week before the training intensive, that Rupert had been sold to someone unknown to me, two weeks after I had landed in the States. He had been transported to France where I would have no chance of a reunion. With the relocation, I was already feeling lost at sea. We had been in the country for about two months and I was feeling homesick for my friends, family, and familiarity. Hearing the news about Rupert left me feeling like I had been thrown overboard.

As we walked out to the corral, we were instructed to go and meet the herd and spend time with the horse we felt most drawn to. Not wanting to bring myself into the herd with any pretense, simply to go through the motions to satisfy the task given, I positioned myself along the fence line with my back against the fence. I looked out across the corral at the 15 or so horses who had lifted their heads from grazing at the sight of 10 people walking into their space. I saw a group of my fellow trainees walking up to a horse at the far end of the corral.

Suddenly, this mare lifted her head above the group of people in front of her and began to push her way through the group. She whinnied as she pointed her ears directly at me and trotted across the corral with purpose. Stopping in front of me, she sniffed, and bowed her head and placed her forehead on my chest. I was completely taken aback by her actions, but stood still and breathed deeply. The rest of the group faded into the background. Something about this interaction held meaning for me, but I wasn't yet sure what that was. I was aware of a deep settling in my body and a feeling of familiarity that I couldn't explain. The mare lifted her head and looked at me. I saw my reflection in her bright, clear eyes. The moment seemed to last forever.

As it happened, while I was stood in awe of this horse whom I felt had so deliberately chosen to stand with me, the owner of the facility walked by the fence line behind me. "I see you've met Dina," she said. "Yes. Apparently she really wanted to meet me," I replied. "I don't think I've seen a horse with this kind of marking in the States before. What breed is she? Back home, we'd call her a Gypsy Cob, but I didn't think you had them here," I asked. "Well, we call them Gypsy Vanners here, but this one is a Gypsy Cob, for sure," she replied, "She was imported from England. She's only been here about two months."

I was stunned. I looked back at Dina and began to cry. I truly believed that somehow, this majestic mare had felt my anguish of being in a foreign land, and my grief for my pony. Somehow, she had sought me out amongst the group of participants, the only English person. Perhaps she resonated with the energy I brought into the corral. Perhaps she recognized my homesickness. Somehow, not only did she notice me, but she had deliberately sought me out.

In my mind, I rationalized that she could not have known that we shared a common home; I had not even uttered a word, so it wasn't as though she recognized my accent! And yet, here she was, standing before me with her open heart and gentle eyes, welcoming me into her space and enveloping me with her presence. That moment was truly an I-Thou encounter with another being. She saw me fully, and I met her in that that space between us with gratitude.

This chapter outlines the core themes of how the theoretical foundations can be translated into clinical practice. From the existing literature on EFPL, theories on why and how it works center around these main themes: Projection/Mirroring, Attachment, and Groundwork versus Mounted Work.

PROJECTION/MIRRORING

There exists a general consensus within the EFPL community of why horses are such powerful partners in this work. People often refer to the horses as "mirrors" in the therapeutic and learning process, to refer to their ability to show us what we are feeling by mirroring our behaviors and emotions. Whilst on the one hand, we can acknowledge that these magnificent animals are highly sensitive, intuitive, and wise beings with much to teach us, there is a tendency to reduce them into blank screens for projection. This is both inaccurate and unfair on our equine partners, because the moment that we lose sight of them as a sentient being in their own right, is the moment we lose sight of the relationship. To focus only on their capacity to teach us about ourselves through a projective lens, diminishes the powerful insights we might gain. As leading EFP practitioner and author Shannon Knapp asserts, the horses are "more than a mirror." At the Human-Equine Relational Development (HERD) Institute, we believe that horses offer a relational presence that is often missing from our clients' lives, and it is their individual way of responding to our clients that bring about healing. They are equal partners in the process and not a tool to be used simply to project our feelings onto.

Critics and/or skeptics of EFPL may well question how we know that the horse is offering acceptance and nonjudgment in their way of relating with us, and in fact place the emphasis of the work within the theoretical confines of projection on the client's part. How do we know that the *I-Thou* encounter between horse and client is not simply of the client's fantasy? How do we know if the horse is approaching the client with that commitment to engage?

These are valid questions and worthy of exploration. For this, we return to our philosophical foundations.

In the movement between *I-Thou* and *I-It* modes of relating, Buber called attention to the moment when we retreat into our own experience to the exclusion of the other, so that in our experience, the other becomes a part of our self and does not embody otherness with which to relate. From a theoretical perspective, this could be seen as a form of projection and/or disconnection from the relationship. Projection is viewed as two distinct parts. The first refers to the process by which we attribute to the environment aspects of ourselves that are out of our awareness or disowned, and the second refers to the process whereby the disowned aspect is attributed to objects or persons in the environment, and then experienced as directed *toward* ourselves. Philippson believed that projection is an unavoidable part of being alive in the world, and this process naturally becomes a part of the therapeutic process in the form of transference.

There are a multitude of differing opinions about the definition, role, and validity of the concept of transference in psychotherapy literature. From a psychoanalytic perspective, transference refers specifically to attributes of a significant other being projected onto the therapist from the client and was originally given by Freud as a "hypothetical process whereby various emotions and attitudinal reactions from the client's past intruded on the present therapeutic relationship." As such, transference is an integral ingredient to the psychoanalytical process and was traditionally fostered through adhering to a strict code of non-disclosure and making available a blank screen of the therapist, upon which the client could project his past experience. In contrast, from Existential-Humanistic and Gestalt perspectives, transference and projection are viewed as ways in which individuals make sense of their field, recreating in the here-and-now what occurred in the there-and-then. When the past is recreated often enough, it becomes the client's life story. Since we are working within a holistic and relational model, rather than viewing transference as something to be interpreted and encouraged in the therapeutic environment, we must acknowledge that the therapist's action/reaction cannot be separated from the client's experience, so that whatever occurs in the therapy process is considered to be cocreated. This allows us to acknowledge our part in the relationship rather than accentuating a power differential within the therapeutic encounter by ascribing projection and transference as solely belonging to the client. Within the context of the HERD approach, this cocreated experience occurs between the client, horse(s) and therapist, always situated within an environment of continuous flow between the *I-Thou* and *I-It*.

Within the HERD approach, it is encouraged for the horses to be at liberty during a session. Whether this is in a stall, paddock, or arena, it is important for the horses to feel that they are able to come and go as they please. Obviously, this is limited within the confines of a stall, but as long as the horse is not tied in place, they can still choose to turn away and disengage.

By engaging with the experience of the horses, and accepting that they are beings with their own agency, it would be possible to surmise that the horses would move away from the client and/or not pay attention to them if they were not actively engaged in the interaction. Often, for clients, it is the horse's willingness to stay with them whilst they are struggling with difficult feelings that acts as confirmation of the horse's acceptance of them. Theoretically, any projection from the client onto the horse would be part of the constant flow between an *I-Thou* and *I-It* encounter, and taken as part of the cocreated experience between them. This co-created perspective gives support to the clients' possible feelings of their need for intimacy, connection, and compassion in relationship with the horse. In this way, the horse is attuned to the client's feelings and responding to them as another being in their own right and not simply acting as a mirror to the client's feelings.

ATTACHMENT

Including horses into the therapeutic space does not mean a negation of the therapist-client relationship. Instead, EFP relies not only on the therapeutic relationship with the practitioner, but is made more powerful by the client's attachment to the horse. This opportunity for nurturing a healthier attachment process can also be viewed through a traditional attachment theory concept referred to as *holding*. There are three aspects of holding within EFP: the physical sensation of being held while on horseback; the natural setting within a horse barn providing a nonthreatening environment; and the acceptance and non-judgmental nature of the horses. These three elements combine to offer clients the secure base and sanctuary necessary for healthy attachment. In this way, horses provide a nonjudgmental presence that may be experienced as the unconditional love that fosters secure attachment, and thereby offer psychological healing.

GROUNDWORK

Horses respond to shifts in energetic intention and communicate within the herd through their ability to regulate their own life energy, or *chi*. When watching a herd of horses in the pasture, we can witness the directed movements of the herd through this energetic intention from one horse to another. The nonverbal behaviors exhibited by horses within the herd are often transferred to humans when they enter into their environment and this offers clients an experiential process of immediate biofeedback on their own life energy and intentions.

Chi is not only energy that we feel internally and from others, but an all-encompassing life force that also indicates a sense of flow and directionality, but according to Hamilton, it also relates to "the vitality of breathing and implies a concept of fundamental vigor, potency, or energetic activity." Regulation of our personal energy is an important aspect of becoming embodied, as our energetic flow can be impacted by our internal emotions and external environment. Emotions in this context can be defined as "energy-in-motion" that flow through our body and influences the organic functioning of our self. When placed in the context of an embodied approach to psychotherapy, the therapist's task is to support clients to attune to their emotions through energetic awareness.

Working with horses through groundwork offers clients a powerful insight into their awareness of their own energetic power and intentions and increases their ability to regulate their energy. The HERD approach incorporates groundwork into sessions from a relational perspective of supporting clients to approach and engage with horses through grooming, petting, walking with, and/or breathing with their equine partners. For horses, breathing, sniffing, and feeling with their whiskers are ways of communicating their interest and/or fears. Hamilton expressed the belief that, with horses, "intention begins with inspiration," so that breathing with a horse is an intentionally relational activity that both centers and connects clients with their equine partners. The physiology of intentional deep breathing combines the compression of abdominal organs with an increase of oxygen delivery to the brain that signals the parasympathetic nervous system to slow the heart rate, relax the body, and disengage the amygdala response of fight or flight. When clients are invited to lean against the belly of a horse to breathe with the animal, feeling the rise and fall of the horse's breath with the client's own breath not only fosters the relationship between the horse and the client, but also acts as an embodied reminder of preverbal attachment patterns.

A Word About Working With Trauma

Clients might be invited to pet or groom the horses in order to begin the process of increasing his/her body awareness through physical contact and to further develop a relationship with the horse. Since physical touch precipitates the release of oxytocin and acts as a preverbal method of communication, it allows for a deeper embodied experience for clients. Furthermore, the actual bodily experience of physical contact between the horse and the client becomes an embedded neurological process that reactivates the neuronal pathways for a positive experience of physical touch. This can provide clients with a history of abuse and trauma a safe and restorative avenue towards rehabilitating their experiences of physical touch and intimacy.

MOUNTED WORK

The HERD approach offers an embodied multisensory experience that affects the client's sensory, neurological, psychological, and social processing patterns, as contact with horses can stimulate physiological, psychological, and social responses. During a mounted session, clients are encouraged to use verbal commands as well as body cues that incorporate the movement of seat, leg, and hands. At different gaits, the horse provides different movement patterns and sensory input to the client. While the HERD approach is a distinct therapeutic modality from that of therapeutic riding, it is useful to consider the theories from this discipline as it pertains to mounted work within a session.

Since the gait of the horse is a three-dimensional movement that incorporates longitudinal, lateral, and posterior/anterior motions, a client riding the horse will experience these movements through their pelvis. The movement of the pelvis is not only translated upward along the spine, which stimulates the nervous system, but also impacts the rider's hip joints and legs with movements of adduction/abduction, internal/external rotation, and flexion/extension. In conjunction with these movements, the rider is also stretching the hips and legs around the barrel of the horse. In instances where the client is riding bareback, that is, without a saddle, there is the additional benefit of feeling the warmth of the horse through the legs and seat, which increases circulation to aid the stretching muscles. The three-dimensional movement produced through the gait of the horse is an important element in the HERD approach. Whilst the mechanics of movement are the same in all horses, their conformations (or builds) are different which impacts their movement patterns. In other words, some horses have longer strides at the walk and produce a smoother gait, and some horses walk with a bounce in their step. Similarly, one horse may have a bouncy trot with plenty of impulsion/energy longitudinally, whereas another may have more lateral movement and feel smoother to ride. These differences in movement will have a direct impact on the level of stimuli that the rider experiences in the saddle, which may elicit different emotional responses depending on the client.

During a mounted session, clients will experience an increase in body awareness through bi-lateral coordination, spatial perception, motor planning and control skills, as well as an increase in tactile, vestibular, and proprioceptive senses. Linking this to body-psychotherapies literature on movement and the release of trauma, the movement of the horse helps to facilitate the re-integration of the bodymind. The release of endorphins and oxytocin as a result of physical exercise and contact with the horse can increase a client's sense of self through building confidence and feelings of well being. Combined with the relationship that is built between the client and the horse, this process can create not only an embodied relational shift for clients in their experience of themselves, but also, may illuminate through the power of metaphor the way clients engage in relationships with others in their lives.

In conducting a session using the HERD approach, the aim is not for the therapist to make meaning for the client about what is happening moment to moment during the session. Instead, the focus is for the client to attune to his or her own embodied experience and allow the meaning to surface. This applies also to leaving the horses to engage with the client in such a way to support the client to find meaning of their interactions, without the therapist's interpretations of the horse's actions or behaviors. The emphasis throughout the session is on the interaction between the horse(s), client(s), and therapist, where horses become co-facilitators. Exceptions to this would be in the event of issues of safety. We will discuss safety and ethics next. Since the HERD approach is an embodied process at its core, it is an effective treatment modality for a wide range of clients (see case studies).

Part II

Chapter 6

Ethical Practice in EFPL

Veronica Lac and Elisabeth Crabtree

Professional ethics is of utmost importance in any environment when working with a vulnerable population. Social workers, counselors, and psychologists all have their own professional codes of ethics mandated by their National or State licensing boards, professional memberships, and/or agencies that they must adhere to for continued accreditation and membership. Breaches of ethical conduct result in penalties and/or disqualification from practice. Likewise, in educational settings, there are codes of practice that govern the way that students are treated. This is particularly true when working with students with special needs. The International Coach Federation outlines a code of ethics that member practitioners must follow, and organizational coaches within corporations may have internal regulations that oversee their scope of practice. All of these are an essential component to maintain safety for our clients and uphold credibility for our professions.

Given that Equine-Facilitated Psychotherapy and Learning (EFPL) practitioners come from all walks of life, and are already familiar with these requirements, it should come as no surprise that additional considerations must be incorporated when bringing clients into contact with horses. The Human-Equine Relational Development (HERD) Institute Codes of Ethics and Professional Practice is based on a foundation of Existential-Humanistic principles, and strives to provide practitioners with clear guidelines on horse-human interactions, as a way of holding our members to the highest of standards.

While the full HERD Institute Codes of Ethics and Professional Practice can be found on our website and in our student handbooks, below are excerpts that highlight our expectations of working with clients and equines. This is followed by a more in-depth discussion of specific elements within the codes.

Equine-Facilitated Psychotherapy and Learning. DOI: http://dx.doi.org/10.1016/B978-0-12-812601-1.00006-7

THE PROFESSIONAL RELATIONSHIP

a. With Clients:
  I. HERD Members will respect the dignity, worth and uniqueness of clients and protect the welfare and safety of the client.
  II. HERD Members aim to promote increased awareness, encourage self-support and facilitate the self-development and autonomy of clients with a view to increasing the range of choices available to them, together with their ability/willingness to accept responsibility for the decisions they make.
  III. HERD Members are responsible for working in ways that enhance their client's sense of empowerment, their capacity to become self-supporting, their ability to make creative choices and changes in response to their evolving needs, circumstances, values and beliefs.
  IV. HERD Members will be respectful of their client's age, health, gender, sexuality, religion, ethnic group, social context, and any other significant aspects of their life.
  V. HERD Members must recognize the importance of a good relationship for effective therapy, be cognizant of the power, and influence this responsibility gives them. The Member must act in a manner consistent with this recognition and not exploit any client financially, sexually, or emotionally for his or her own personal advantage or their own needs.
  VI. The HERD Institute believes that a sexual relationship with a client is exploitative. Sexual harassment in the form of deliberate or repeated comments, gestures, or physical contacts of a sexual nature that are, or could be, considered offensive by the client, are unethical.
b. With Equine Partners. . ..
  I. HERD Members will respect the dignity, worth, and uniqueness of each horse and will protect the welfare and safety of each horse.
  II. HERD Members will hold the human-equine relationship as a central concern in the EFPL work, as well as daily interactions, training and riding.
  III. HERD Members will work with a compassionate and consistent approach in regards to their equine partners.
  IV. The overall health and care of the horse is essential, this includes the housing, nutrition, general health, hoof care, and physical and emotional well being of the horse.
  V. The HERD Institute believes that the physical and emotional well being of equine partners is an essential element of the EFPL process. Members must recognize the impact that the work may have on the horses they partner with and be mindful of the responsibility of providing the horses due care and consideration when asking them to work in this way.

VI. HERD Members will neither allow, nor condone, the abuse of horses by drugging, letting of blood, soring, or any other inhumane tactic, and will report anyone using these tactics. This includes the unnecessary restraint of horses for punishment and/or discipline.

VII. HERD Members shall respect the integrity and well being of their equine partners whether owned, leased, or loaned.

VIII. HERD Members must be trained in horsemanship skills to a level that satisfies the HERD training requirements.

IX. HERD Members must demonstrate continued professional development in horsemanship skills as outlined in the Student Handbook.

X. In professional practice, HERD Members must be familiar with the horses they are working with. They must understand the horses' place in the herd, their temperament, level of training, ground manners, physical strengths and weaknesses, and their ability to tolerate people who are inexperienced around horses.

Confidentiality

I. Confidentiality is intrinsic to good practice. All exchanges between HERD Members and clients must be regarded as confidential. HERD Members must abide by their professional Codes of Ethics within their scope of practice. When a Member wishes to use specific information gained during work with a client—in a lecture or publication, the client's permission should be obtained and anonymity preserved. Clients should be informed that they have a right to withdraw consent at any time.

Client Safety

I. HERD Members must take all reasonable steps to protect clients from physical or psychological harm during any EFPL session. This includes safety in working with horses, and the maintenance of safe facilities, equipment, and tack.

II. HERD Members must only place clients on a horse when:
- HERD Members must prepare clients on horse safety issues prior to introducing them to the herd, arena, or around a tied horse.
- The client is wearing a properly fitted helmet, suitable footwear, and appropriate attire.
- The client has been briefed on how to mount the horse.
- All potential risks have been clearly and accurately explained to the client verbally, and a written consent form has been signed.

Continued Development

I. HERD Members will continually monitor their own professional strengths and limitations and will seek to improve through ongoing education and training.

II. We believe that continued education in all areas regarding therapy and horsemanship is essential to all HERD Members and the safety of their clients.

DISCUSSION ON SAFETY AND ETHICS

In relation to EFPL, both safety and ethics are such broad and far-reaching topics that they could each have entire books devoted to them. This discussion outlines some of the basic considerations pertaining to The HERD Institute Codes of Ethics and Professional Practice of which practitioners should be aware. Safety includes the safety of all horses and humans, both physically and emotionally.

THE HERD SAFETY PROTOCOL

Prior to any interaction with the horses, clients must be informed of the inherent risks associated with working with equines. This includes signing liability waivers, and an explanation of how to keep oneself safe around horses. The format we utilize begins with checking in with signing liability documents as soon as (first time) clients arrive at the barn. This is followed by a quick overview and/or review of horse safety. Finally, we utilize a version of Barbara Rector's Adventures in Awareness process of repeating the safety agreement with our participants.

The safety agreement states that, "I agree to be responsible for myself in this session, and thereby contribute to the safety of others in the group."

The verbalization of this allows participants to take ownership of their actions, thoughts, and feelings as the session unfolds, and also calls attention to their physical being and safety.

SAFETY AROUND HORSES

Many of our participants may never have had any previous interaction with horses. Therefore, it is imperative that we discuss basic safety before they approach our horses. Although we ask everyone to take responsibility for their own safety (and thus contribute to the safety of the group), they can only do so within the limitations of their knowledge of the dangers. It is our responsibility to highlight the specific risks of working around horses. It is essential that we do not assume their understanding of what it takes to keep themselves physically safe. The safety agreement is always followed by the emphasis that if there is a situation where the facilitators deem that safety is of concern, we may step in and physically intervene on the client's behalf. This may or may not include physically pulling/pushing/moving client out of harms way.

The HERD Safety Protocol also includes an explanation of the basic horse safety rules in the following manner:

Feet—If a horse steps on our foot, our natural reaction is to try to pull our foot away. Given the relative weight of a horse, this does not work. Instead, because horses respond to pressure, we need to push against the horse so that it moves away and takes it foot off ours.

Vision—Horses, being prey animals, have their eyes located on either side of their head. As such, they have a very wide range of vision, most of which is monocular. However, they have two major blind spots in their field of vision—immediately in front of them and behind them (see Fig. 6.1). It is important that we explain this and how we can safely approach and move around the horses.

Startle response—As we have already mentioned, horses are prey animals and, as such, are always alert to danger. As a result, they are very sensitive to sudden movements or sounds and will startle and/or flee. Horses can move very quickly and there is always a risk of someone being knocked over or crushed by a startled horse.

We need to explain this in our safety protocol and also ask that any small children be supervised. Generally, we would also want to prohibit any clients' animals at our facility.

Leading horses—When our clients are working directly with the horses, we need to identify specific safety issues, such as safe tying or grooming

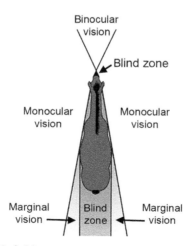

FIGURE 6.1 Equine field of vision.

techniques, and the safe handling of lead ropes. Most importantly, we need to draw attention to not wrapping lead ropes around their hands, or dragging on the ground.

Attire—We must require that our clients wear sensible, safe clothing, and footwear that is appropriate for working around horses. Open sandals or flip-flops are never permitted. No jewelry or accessories that could become entangled in tack or equipment should be worn. If mounted work is being introduced, participants must wear well-fitted, approved riding helmets, regardless of age.

A SAFE THERAPEUTIC RELATIONSHIP

Emotional safety in EFPL is of paramount importance, particularly when there has historically been a muddying of waters regarding scope of practice. It is absolutely essential for EFL practitioners, in particular, to be clear about their level of training and scope of practice, so as not to expose clients to any undue emotional distress without appropriate supports. As EFP practitioners, emotional safety encompasses all the usual requirements of any licensed mental health professional, including the maintenance of confidentiality, record keeping, and inherent risk practices.

Often, EFP practitioners will work in an adjunct treatment capacity in support of a primary therapist. In this instance, it is important to obtain permission from the clients to share treatment and progress information with the therapist. Their primary therapist must also obtain agreement from the clients in order to inform you on the client's presenting issues, and/or to update you on their progress. If working within a multidisciplinary team, such as an outpatient clinic, it is essential that the client contract includes an agency disclosure form in order for the team to share information.

It is imperative that notes are recorded after each session with clients. These notes should identify the client, the date, and duration of the session. They should be signed by the practitioner and record his/her credentials. There are several formal formats for taking notes, including the SOAP system and the DAP system. The SOAP (Subjective, Objective, Assessment, and Plan) system allows practitioners to include their subjective responses to the client and the session. The DAP system is more simplistic and only includes observable data. When used within the context of EFP, the SOAP system provides more leeway to include a more holistic perspective, including the therapist's feelings about the how the horses and clients are interacting with each other. Regardless of the form of note taking used, as with the horses, the "as much as necessary and as little as possible" maxim applies.

These notes will serve as a useful *aide mémoire* for future sessions. Notes should be considered highly confidential, not shared with anyone, and kept in a double-locked repository. As a licensed mental health professional, it is important to continue to do your own personal work and find a suitable supervisor who is willing to work with you. As an EFP practitioner, this should be someone with experience in equine-facilitated approaches, as they will more fully understand the unique issues and challenges of EFP.

THE ROLE OF ASSISTANTS

If we work mostly with individuals, couples, or families, with only one or two horses, it is quite possible that we will be able to work without additional help—much as we would conduct our work in an office environment. However, we might decide to include assistants in our work, especially if we are working with larger groups and/or multiple horses.

Assistants may take on specific roles, such as adjuvant, equine support, or cofacilitator. Whatever role they are fulfilling, assistants must be given appropriate training for that role, and understand what is expected of them.

Cofacilitator

Particularly when working with large groups, it may be necessary to have additional qualified therapists, trainers, or educators working with us. If so, we will need to fully discuss the format of the session(s) and clarify the role and responsibilities of each professional. As the facilitators, this dynamic must be a strong model of trust, boundaries, and clear communication. Participants will take their lead from the facilitation team as to how safe the group feels to them. A solid working partnership is one that allows for flexibility as well as holding space for what might emerge.

Equine Support Staff

Some EFP/EFL models recommend or require the inclusion of an "Equine Specialist" in the work, and training and certifications are available for this specific role. Within the HERD approach to EFPL, the therapist/trainer/educator/coach is dually qualified as an equine professional, so it is not mandatory to include additional equine support staff. If present, the equine support staff serves as the equine expert during equine/human interaction, and is specifically responsible for the health and wellbeing of the horses engaged in the work. Equine support staff are experienced in horsemanship, while also understanding how to work with EFPL practitioners in order to ensure the safety of all.

Adjuvants

While we may not feel that working with an equine support staff fits our program, it is likely that we will need additional help when we are working with larger groups and multiple horses. Adjuvants should be experienced and competent in handling horses, understand the work we are doing, able to assist with logistics and to oversee safety. While it may seem that this role is identical to that of the equine support staff, the emphasis is somewhat different. Adjuvants typically take on a wider scope of duties than equine support staff and may assist with handling horses, fetching equipment, organizing paperwork, or preparing lunch.

Regardless of which type of assistants we include in our work, they must be given adequate training and orientation in order to fulfill their role(s) effectively. All personnel should know, understand, and comply with our codes of ethics, the barn rules, and all relevant emergency information. They should be familiar with the horses with which they will interact and the facility in which they are to work. We must be clear in expressing our requirements and expectations; especially regarding the extent to which we anticipate support staff will directly interact with clients and the process. Additionally, they should be briefed before each session and understand the context, purpose, and focus of the session, in order that they can provide the appropriate assistance, while remaining flexible and responsive to a change of plan, if necessary.

A SAFE PLACE

We have a duty of care to both the humans and horses involved in our work. Additionally, our insurance companies and any applicable "protective" legislation will only support us if we are working in a manner that is not willfully or wantonly negligent with respect to safety.

We must, therefore, ensure that the working environment is free of hazards. Our workspace must be clean, safe, and well maintained at all times. This includes such considerations as:

- Safe footing in our arenas or workspaces
- Ensuring all areas provide adequate lighting and climate control
- Providing secure doors, gates, or barriers where appropriate
- Keeping tack and equipment clean and in good repair and inspecting it before use
- Maintaining a clean environment
- Ensuring no hazards exist such as loose boards, debris underfoot, etc.

The owner of a facility is also responsible for ensuring that:

- Appropriate signage is legible.
- All exits and emergency exits are clearly marked and unlocked.
- All aisles and walkways are clear and free of obstructions.
- Steps are kept clear of trip hazards and snow or ice.
- Fire-suppression equipment is suitably positioned, clearly marked, and regularly inspected.

- First aid supplies (human and horse) are readily accessible, labeled, and stocked.
- All utilities are in good repair—including electrical wiring and switches.
- Restroom facilities are clean, well maintained, accessible, and marked.
- Emergency evacuation plans/routes are clearly posted.
- Emergency muster point(s) are clearly marked.
- Emergency contact information is prominently displayed, including the exact location for responders.
- All restricted substances are clearly marked and appropriately secured.
- MSDS sheets are readily accessible and identified, if appropriate.
- Any restricted areas are clearly marked.
- Horses and vehicles are segregated—with parking areas clearly defined and marked.
- Facility rules and/or policies are prominently displayed. These may include rules around appropriate attire, the handling and feeding of horses, cleaning, securing equipment and implements, securing gates and barriers, prohibition or control of small children and animals, noise, speed limits, and restricted areas.

LEVELING THE PLAYING FIELD: A PLACE IN THE HERD

By Veronica Lac, PhD

In any discussion on ethics, it is essential to give consideration to issues of diversity. By this, I mean for practitioners to pay *active* attention and be sensitive to differences in socioeconomic, racial, ethnic, educational, class, gender, sexuality, physical, and neurodiversity. It is not enough to pay lip service to these concepts from a majority perspective. Practitioners must possess the self-awareness and motivation to seek out their own blind spots in these issues so that they can truly provide an inclusive environment, without inadvertently alienating their clients.

I used to live in a Central Ohio suburb. It is the kind of place where kids play on the street in front of their homes while dogs lie on front porches watching the world go by and the neighbors all know each other by name. On a summer evening, the smell of steaks cooking on outdoor grills and freshly cut grass would waft through the air. The white picket fences, traditional mailboxes, and manicured lawns that surrounded me are a symbol of privilege and a testament to achieving the American Dream. It's the Hollywood version of suburban America that I grew up watching in movies and TV shows in England.

I imagine that it would be possible to live a whole lifetime in this bubble and exist within a 10-minute driving radius from this community. Everything I needed and everyone I knew in the area lived within that distance. So I could go to work, walk my dogs around the neighborhood, visit friends in

the area, do my grocery shopping, and go to the barn all without acknowledging that there was a bigger, wider, *different* world beyond those suburban
streets.

While a part of me felt like I belonged in this homogenous bubble, I also
knew that I didn't.

I know what it is like to be different. I know what it means to not look,
sound, and feel the same as those around me. I'm so familiar and sensitive
to issues of diversity it's like I embody them on a cellular level. I work with
disadvantaged youths and those with cognitive, emotional, and physical challenges. I am passionate about social equality, human and civil rights, and
have been exposed to enough injustice to know that my privileged world
within the white picket fences was not representative of the world at large.
But I wonder how I might feel about diversity issues if I hadn't had those
experiences? I wonder what it might be like to not be aware of my privi-
leges? How easy would it be to turn a blind eye to those that don't have
them?

Often, discussions about diversity lead to confrontations and feelings of
hurt, anger, and betrayal. Well-intentioned friends and colleagues can step
onto a minefield of microaggressions; unknowingly participating in the rein-
forcement of race, ethnic, gender, sexuality, and socioeconomic status stereo-
types. We place each other into an "us" or "them" dichotomy and lose sight
of our connections with each other. These experiences make it difficult to
continue to engage in these discussions, however, important they may be. As
therapists, teachers, parents, and leaders in our communities, how can we
learn to model inclusiveness in order to keep the dialogue alive?

As an EFPL practitioner I, naturally, spend a lot of time both professionally and personally, with these majestic animals observing their behaviors and how they interact with each other. I've worked with different
breeds of horses in different countries, different facilities, and different riding disciplines. I used to board my horse at a facility with a diverse range of
horses that included off-the-track thoroughbreds, dressage, showjumping,
and 3-day-eventing horses through to Western reining, cutting, trail horses,
and regular riding school and 4-H ponies as well as therapeutic riding horses.
Some of the horses came with distinguished bloodlines and heavy price tags,
others were show champions with multiple trophies, or had never competed,
or were rescued from slaughter. The beauty of all this diversity is that while
we might associate the 3-day-eventer horse with his rich, Ivy-League edu-
cated, corporate lawyer owner and the therapeutic riding horse with the nonprofit organization run by volunteers, when the horses are grazing in the
fields with each other none of that is relevant to them.

When people tell me that horses are a great example of how to work with
diversity because they are completely non-judgmental and don't see differences, I become wary. When we assume that being non-judgmental

automatically results in equality, we are missing the point. There's also a danger in thinking that being nonjudgmental means that we don't have to engage in the conversation.

The aim of becoming more competent in working with diversity is not in assuming that everyone is the same, but in acknowledging and addressing differences while staying connected within the relationship.

That's what horses are great models for.

As herd animals, horses rely on each other for survival. The social system within a herd is a highly developed one with defined codes of behavior and customs. While the herd is hierarchical, respect is not gained through size or strength of muscle, nor through the number of winning trophies achieved or pedigree breeding and physical attributes. Their monetary value and accolades are inconsequential in the herd because they do not contribute to the survival of the herd. Respect within the herd is manifested in the ability to lead others to safety while modeling clear boundaries and maintaining harmony. Relationships are formed where every member plays a vital role to ensure cohesion, safety, and harmony within the herd. When differences present themselves through changes in the herd as members come and go or in conflicts with each other, horses respond by addressing the differences in an inclusive way with the benefit of the whole herd in mind. The momentary discomfort in addressing the difference is outweighed by maintaining the relationships between members and thus ensuring the safety of the herd.

As therapists, coaches, educators and trainers, we must value the practice of discovering our blind spots in order to broaden our perspectives. By owning our limitations, we can deepen our relationships with clients. Talking about diversity challenges us to sit with discomfort and raises our awareness about what we take for granted. It is about examining our assumptions and exploring how we can all take responsibility for addressing differences, create a more inclusive society, and find ways of leveling the playing field. By staying connected in the difficult dialogues, perhaps we can each find our place in the herd in a more harmonious way.

ETHICS OF WORKING WITH HORSES

At the HERD Institute, we subscribe to the Compassionate Equestrian principles of horsemanship. These 25 principles were developed by Dr. Allen Schoen and Susan Gordon, who offer in their book, *The Compassionate Equestrian*, a way of working with horses that honors the horse as a sentient being. Based on both art and science, the authors place compassion and empathy at the core of their teachings to develop meaningful partnerships with their horses. The 25 principles cover all aspects of care and consideration for our equine partners, highlighting the importance of maintaining a humane and gentle approach to any interactions, embracing a holistic and integrative approach to equine health care. By instilling a foundation of mindfulness and self-awareness to all interactions with our horses, the Compassionate Equestrian approach is a natural fit with the philosophies of the HERD approach to EFPL. At the heart of their message, is the maxim that we should treat our horses as we would wish to be treated ourselves, with respect, dignity, and compassion.

As indicated in the HERD Codes of Ethics and Professional Practice, this approach is fundamental in our philosophy. It is essential for practitioners to remember that we enter into this way of working holding the belief that horses are healers. However, many of the horses we work with did not necessarily have a choice where they ended up. For this reason, we advocate that we must pay attention to the emotional well being of our horses in doing this work, and offer them the choice to engage or not, if at all possible. This means ideally working at liberty so that horses can come and go as they please, and engage with clients in their own way, at their own pace, should they choose to do so. We must recognize the impact that the work may have on the horses, being mindful to provide the horses due care and consideration. Ideally, we will be familiar with the horses we are working with. We will understand the horses' place in the herd, their temperament, level of training, ground manners, physical strengths and weaknesses, and their ability to tolerate people who are inexperienced around horses.

Leading on from this, in addition to the emotional well being of our horses, their overall health and care is of utmost importance. This includes the housing, nutrition, general health, and foot care. All tack and equipment used should be appropriate, well fitted, clean and in good condition, such that it is safe, and causes neither physical nor emotional distress to the horses. Proper saddle fitting is crucial if mounted work is to be included. Bridles with bits should be avoided for inexperienced riders, and substituted with the use of halters and snap on reins.

Finally, the HERD Institute will not allow or condone its members to abuse horses in any way. No horse should be asked to perform beyond their capabilities, particularly with respect to the weight of riders during mounted work. Weight limits should be calculated for each horse in the herd. A general rule of thumb would be to 20% of the horse's weight. This should include tack in the overall weight load, particularly as Western saddles may weigh upward of 30 lbs. We must cease working with a horse immediately if it appears to be in pain or distress.

The ethical principles outlined above are at the core of the HERD approach. This will be evident in the following chapters as we outline the HERD approach to EFPL, and in the case study examples. It is our hope that by emphasizing this compassionate way of relating to our equine partners that it becomes a way-of-being for the HERD practitioner, and thus makes a positive contribution to the world around them.

HORSEMANSHIP DEVELOPMENT

With regard to horsemanship, the learning process never ends. In line with the HERD Model's subscription to the 25 Principles of Compassionate Equestrians, as a way of supporting the HERD Institute's codes of ethics and professional practice, practitioners must be cognizant of the holistic health and welfare of their equine partners by demonstrating their knowledge in the following areas:

Riding & Groundwork
Selection & Care of Tack & Equipment
Horse Behavior & Communication
Equine Nutrition
Herd Dynamics
Stable & Pasture Management
Equine Health & First Aid
Hoof Care

At the HERD Institute, the training program incorporates all of the above elements to some degree. However, it is important for students to find their own style of working with horses that compliments the training, so supplemental training in specific horsemanship and/or equine studies is encouraged. While some EFPL practitioners come with extensive horsemanship experience, others may be approaching the work from a mental health professional and/or educator/coach/trainer background and just beginning to incorporate horses into their work. For this reason, we advocate a personalized development plan for students to assess, integrate, and support their existing horsemanship knowledge and skills. Additionally, while horseback riding techniques are not necessary to conduct the work, it is advisable for practitioners to have a basic understanding of the feel of being on horseback in all gaits, horse conformation, and the impact this has on equine biomechanics, and the subsequent impact on the rider. It is highly discouraged for practitioners to ask clients to experiment with someone on horseback without having experienced the activity or movement themselves.

HORSE SUITABILITY

Every horse has the potential to teach us something. While this is true for those of us who have been around horses long enough to generally know how to keep ourselves safe and work with them within our capabilities, it takes a special kind of horse to work in an EFPL environment. Many horses become "therapy" horses by chance and circumstances, and have helped support healing for a wide variety of clients. Many of them arrive with histories of trauma themselves, and have much to offer our clients in terms of trauma recovery. However, it is important to ensure that our clients are not exposed to unnecessary risks that come with being in contact with horses that are unfamiliar with what is expected of them, and/or unprepared for the work we do. While we are not advocating for horses to be trained to do certain tasks or activities, there are a number of factors that need to be considered when preparing a horse to work with our clients.

Essential to our clients' safety is the practitioner's knowledge of the horses that they are partnering with. Aside from issues mentioned previously with regards to knowledge of the horses in terms of logistical planning, that is, whether a horse can be tied/cross-tied, which horses they can/cannot be turned out with, and if conducting mounted work, whether they can be ridden or not, and their weight limits, we must also be cognizant of the horses' window of tolerance for various activities.

Prior to working with a horse, we need to assess the following:

- We understand that horses are prey animals and they are apt to react suddenly to unfamiliar sights/sounds/touch. Is the horse steady enough to withstand unexpected situations without endangering those around them?
- How does the horse react around people? Are they tolerant of having multiple people surrounding them? How do they react to being touched and groomed? To having their feet picked up? How do they respond to an inexperienced person leading them?
- If mounted work is involved, are they familiar with being ridden bareback? Are they beginner safe? How sensitive are they to a rider's seat and leg aides?
- If props are being used in the arena, have the horses been exposed to them before? Cones, barrels, ground poles, balls etc. Whatever is being presented to the client, the horse must have been prepared for prior.
- Do the horses have a choice in whether to engage or not?
- What policies are in place to ensure that the horses do not get burn out? Do you know the signs of burn out for the horses you are working with?
- What policies are in place for allowing the horse to release emotion/tensions following a session?

Ultimately, suitability is dependent on the practitioner's knowledge, skills, and diligence in ensuring that their equine partners are ready to embark on working in this way. Our aim is not to train the horses to respond to our clients in any particular way, but to allow them to bring themselves authentically into the relationship. This can only happen if their needs are being met physically and emotionally outside of the sessions. A horse with a sore back being offered for bareback activities would not be conducive to the healing or safety of our clients. A horse that is tender footed may not be willing/able to accompany our clients on an in-hand trail walk on gravel footing. A horse with a history of trauma at the hands of humans, and who has not had the chance to release and recalibrate from it, may not be suitable for a highly anxious client that is afraid of unpredictability. These considerations must be at the forefront of the practitioner's mind before entering into the work.

In line with the philosophy and theory of practice of the HERD approach to EFPL, we advocate for a holistic approach to working with our horses to prepare them for the work. Of course, there will be much that we cannot foresee, and as with anything with horses, unpredictability is always present. However, it is our job to minimize any potential hazards for our clients. In this way, we can allow the process to unfold and trust that our horses are bringing themselves into each encounter having had their needs met. In turn, this allows them to meet our clients fully and authentically.

Chapter 7

The HERD Model of Equine-Facilitated Psychotherapy

The HERD Model of Equine-Facilitated Psychotherapy (EFP) emerged from my foundations as a Gestalt therapist, and through my research during my doctoral program on the embodied experiences of participants during EFP sessions. The HERD Model follows the definitions outlined previously regarding the licensing requirements of the EFP practitioner. However, the practitioner may be dually qualified as both the therapist and the equine support staff. Indeed, it is our belief that the process necessitates the therapist to also have an in-depth understanding of the equine knowledge and skills found in an equine specialist. The therapist, however, may choose to work with an equine support staff if so desired. This is particularly encouraged when working with groups in order to maintain safety for both horses and humans during a session. The HERD Model of EFP is applicable for working with individuals, couples, families, and groups.

Firmly rooted in the philosophical traditions of phenomenology and I-Thou relating, and integrated with Existential-Humanistic and Gestalt theories, the HERD Model offers students and practitioners a framework for clinical practice. It consists of five stages: Sharing Space, Release and Expand, Deepening, Coming Home, and Integration.

STAGE ONE: SHARING SPACE

When we enter into the herd, our first awareness needs to be centered on our own phenomenal experience of that moment. What am I sensing internally, and how is that impacting my ability to be present with the horses? I usually begin this process by checking in with my breathing, and supporting my client to do the same. How deeply am I breathing? What tensions am I holding in my bodily being? What emotions are beginning to surface as I pay attention to myself? Is my mind wandering to other aspects of my life outside of this present moment? This intentional arrival into the here and now allows me to acknowledge that I am sharing space with another being. As the client begins to notice and verbalize their immediate sensations, I may encourage them to breathe deeper and begin to explore what

Equine-Facilitated Psychotherapy and Learning. DOI: http://dx.doi.org/10.1016/B978-0-12-812601-1.00007-9

entering into the herd feels like to them. Entering the herd may mean stepping into an arena, a stall, or a paddock to be in the presence of one or multiple horses. This will have a different significance for each client and it is the role of the therapist to track these responses. Whether they are familiar with horses or not will have an impact on their reactions to entering the herd. It may be that this is their first session, or they may be regular clients. Again, this will have an impact on their phenomenal experiences. The horse(s) may be at a distance or within close proximity. Regardless of the setup of the facility (more on that in Part 3), these beginning moments of a session require consideration for how we introduce the horse(s) and client into a shared space.

In entering the herd, we are entering into the horses' space. It is important to be respectful of this and I encourage students and clients to observe how horses meet and greet each other. The first interaction between herd members is always a shared breath; they sniff and breathe each other in. It is how they greet humans too.

In my research, participants identified that the beginning moments of establishing a connection with the horses through their breath was a significant moment of awareness. Paying attention to this slowing down and conscious breathing allows clients to begin the process of connecting with himself or herself in an embodied way. As the client focuses on their breath, and the rhythmic breathing of the horse, they may simultaneously begin to touch the horse. This touch will bring about both physiological and psychological shifts. The sensation of warmth through this touch may elicit a sense of both separateness and togetherness, and the awareness of both of them as existential beings, alive together. It may be an act of grounding, both within the client as emotional regulation, and the outward physical support of leaning into the horse, and may be a catalyst in the client's process of being able to pay fuller attention to his/her bodily sensations. These non-verbal experiences lead to a sense of freedom in not having to explain or rationalize the experience through simply being allowed to be present with the horse and/or therapist, sharing space.

Theory: The importance of the breath can be linked to Levine's understanding of the importance of the parasympathetic nervous system, where breathing patterns are indications of the emotional state of the individual, and where conscious, focused breathing can help to alleviate the symptoms of trauma and calm the body. This experience of breathing with the horse is an intentionally relational act. In terms of touch, there has been much research into the physiological benefits of petting a companion animal, providing the embodied comfort that is needed through physical contact by increasing levels of oxytocin that calms and relaxes the body.

Philosophically, this intentional act of sharing space is a direct reflection of Buber's *I-Thou* process of dialogue through shared silence. The act of touching the horse and recognizing it as being in relationship with the other also reflects the origination of Buber's *I-Thou* encounter of his experience with his grandmother's horse. The embodied aliveness that each individual brings into the relationship, creates the "strange kinship" as described by Merleau-Ponty; this is experienced through this joining together as they resonate with one another as "self in relation". Within Gestalt theory, this process of being together can be seen as the experience of inclusive presence in the way that Polster and Polster described as the union of two separate beings joining together while maintaining their sense of separateness.

The role of the HERD practitioner is one of supporting the client to pay attention to what is occurring in the present moment in their embodied being. Through this connection with breath and touch, the client will begin to calm their nervous system and level of arousal, and it is the practitioner's role to create a safe container for the client to experiment with a more grounded state of being. Pat Ogden, somatic psychotherapist and founder of the Sensorimotor Psychotherapy Institute, defines being grounded as the "capacity to direct somatic energy toward the ground and bring awareness to the legs and feet in order to increase the felt sense of a physical base of support." This embodied regulation creates the necessary conditions for the relationships between horse, therapist, and client to develop.

STAGE TWO: RELEASE AND EXPAND

As we enter into any new or renewed relationship, there is always a dance that occurs between how much to lean into the other and how much to hold back. As we negotiate this dance, we become aware of our boundaries, internal stories, and constraints. If, as Mark Rowland suggests, humans are the only animals who believe the stories we tell ourselves, then what stories are we constructing as we enter into relationships? What external rules have we absorbed without question or inherited about how to be in relationship with another? Having experienced shared space, breathing, and touch with the horse(s), how can we now allow ourselves to be seen more fully?

Clients often come into therapy with fixed patterns of behavior (fixed gestalts) that are out of their awareness. These patterns show up in the way that they relate to the therapist and to the horses. Whatever occurs in the here and now, is often a habitual response, and it is in our capacity as the therapist to draw attention to that process. Clients may approach the horses with anticipation and excitement, or they may stand back and wait for the horses to come to them. Whatever their process is, the therapist must maintain a phenomenological stance and active curiosity of what that might mean to the client. Are they holding on to a rule (or introject in Gestalt terms, that is, something that has been integrated into their being without question) about how to behave? Have they already played out in their minds what the horses might think or feel about them, and thereby restrain themselves from further contact? What emotions might be stirring for them as they pay attention to how the horses are interacting with them? Often, clients will come into the space with preconceived ideas about what should or shouldn't happen with the horses. How might that affect the relational process?

This stage of the process centers on the releasing of psychological constriction and the expansion of one's horizons, and is experienced as reaching beyond one's boundaries and the dismantling of barriers. As we release from internalized constraints or rules, and move toward a more integrated experience of our self, we become more aware of the physical sensations of constriction in our body. This leads to a full surrender and letting go of one's "shoulds" in order to be fully present in the moment with the other. In connection with the non-verbal aspect of the embodied experience of sharing space, this release is also felt as an alignment and gathering together of previously fragmented parts of oneself to arrive at a coherent expression, without the need for rationalization and/or justification. In other words, we begin to develop a felt sense of our own authentic presence.

From my research, participants emphasized the relational nature of this stage of the process. By letting go of something internally, we are simultaneously reaching out toward something. This relational nature of the process involves immediate feedback between the client and horse, fosters a connection between client, horse, and therapist, and provides the client with a new experience of being in relationship. This brings with it an embodied sensation of expansion within one self, and forms the beginning of the client's ability to lean into the relationship in a more authentic way. This embodied expansion may extend to a broadening of the client's horizons and an awareness of the interconnectedness with others and his/her environment.

In seeing others and the environment around them more clearly, clients are able to allow others to see them more fully, and begin to offer some transparency in their way of relating to others. This transparency translates into a greater willingness to be open with others, and an expansion by clients of their possibilities of engaging with the world in a more holistic and mindful way, thus creating a softening toward themselves of their own vulnerabilities. It is at once compassionate and confirming, and a reclamation of their sense of self. Reclaiming oneself brings the risk of exposure, so it is in this moment of realization that the client embraces their authenticity. The embodied experience of release and expansion both widens the horizons of clients' perspectives of themselves, while simultaneously unifying their experience of themselves, integrating the fragmented and/or polarized aspects, and reveals more of what was previously kept hidden from others.

This second stage in the HERD Model is crucial in the development of the client's relationship with the horse and therapist. It is in this release and expansion that the client is able to bring themselves more fully into contact and connection with those around them. The role of the HERD practitioner is to notice, moment by moment, the shifts that are happening for the client; tracking their breath and their body movements, paying attention to the process rather than content of what they are bringing, and allowing the client to interact with the horse in their own way. Throughout all of this, we look to the horse's responses to the client's process and maintain a phenomenological stance to allow the clients to make meaning of their experiences for themselves.

Theory: Horses offer a unique and curative medium for clients who otherwise struggle with emotional communication, providing a catalyst for psychological change within the client. The experience of a surrendering of habitually defended ways of encountering others allows clients a moment's pause to relax long held restrictions or introjects. The non-judgmental companionship that horses offer also provides a secure base for attachment. In Gestalt theory, introjects can be defined as the *shoulds* we assimilated in life that constrict our potential for living spontaneously. Additionally, this embodied experience of psychological constriction reflects Merleau-Ponty's view that our body is our perception of being-in-the-world, as well as the Gestalt theory of our felt sense of our lived experience. There is an existential freedom in this moment of experi-ence that still maintains the relationship to others, and forms the move toward an I-Thou moment of contact.

Within the HERD Model, clients are often asked to explore their habitual patterns of behavior by noticing how they are interacting with the horse(s). Clients may be asked to breathe with the horse to match the horse's rhythm by leaning belly-to-belly with the horse. As they breathe with the horse, they may notice the release of physical constrictions, feel into the relationship with the horse, and let go of some of their habitual behaviors and rules of engagement. This relational and embodied process offers the client an expe-rience of a confirming presence from the horse, and engages the process of self-regulation resulting in the feeling of total acceptance. This forms the beginning of an I-Thou meeting between the horse and the client, and the starting point for attachment to occur.

This interconnected aspect of the process can be viewed from a central concept within Gestalt therapy where one's experience of the other changes both parties: it is a cocreated endeavor. The clients' experiences of the horses and their environment also shift their embodied sense of themselves. This occurs as being with horses extracts clients from their intrapersonal domain into a more mindful and interpersonal realm with their whole being. Philippson referred to this embodied experience as living to the full-ness of your skin. There is a sense of wholeness of being, of reoccupying parts of ourselves, hitherto forgotten or hidden. This is reminiscent of Buber's *I-Thou* approach to embodied authenticity of giving oneself fully to the encounter that includes the risk that one takes in choosing to step into relationships.

STAGE THREE: DEEPENING

The willingness to give oneself fully to the encounter brings about the deepening of any relationship. The mutuality found in the connection with the horses allows for clients to experience a feeling of returning to a place of fullness of being; an arrival to a familiar place where one is recognized by self and others, and as such, a sense of belonging. Within this stage of the process, clients will often describe a sense of interconnectedness to the world around them, coupled with the experience of an inner knowing that incorporates listening intently to that which resides within them, and the return to a place where they feel they can trust themselves. This embodied sense of intuition is sometimes accompanied by a physical sensation of sinking deeper into the ground, and is felt as an arrival at a time and place where one can linger while being-in-the-world both individually and collectively with others. This feeling of returning to oneself and belonging to a greater collective is extremely valuable, as it is part of the process of opening oneself up to being seen more fully by others in relationship in order to belong. Ruella Frank refers to this as the moment where "I see you see me. I feel you feel me."

From my research, participants emphasized the unconditional trust that they felt in relationship with the horses, and the feeling of not being able to hide from what they are experiencing in the moment, with the belief that the horses accept them as they are without judgment. This process of deepening in the relationship also incorporates feelings of intentionality and personal agency for clients, as well as gaining a greater sense of integrity in relation to another, which may bring about the confirmation of the inner experience of knowing their own truth and solidifying their sense of themselves. This leads to the potential for clients of the intentional embrace of internal strength and resilience and the ownership of their power. This intentionality may be explored through deliberate movement and the physical act of touching the horses, or in experiencing the solidity of the horse as they breathe together. This solidified sense of self-agency heightens their ability to deepen the relationship in the present moment through their embodied aliveness.

Within the HERD Model, the therapist might support the developing attachment in the client-horse relationship by enhancing the embodied experience through inviting the client to hug, stroke, sniff, or lean into or onto the horse. These sensory experiences allow for the client to surrender their physical selves to another being who is physically and emotionally bearing witness to their journey of relational and self-discovery. The emotional trust and felt sense of safety that this embodied experience brings strengthens the therapeutic alliance between the client and therapist, and allows for the client to open up new ways of being-in-the-world. Clients are often encouraged to move their bodies to bring awareness to their physical being. The physical sensations brought about through the intentional act of moving one's body allow the client to engage in their embodied process and activate the neurological pathways to create the opportunity of experiencing themselves engaging with the world differently. When a ridden component is introduced into a HERD session, it is often with the aim of providing the client a more immediate sense of grounding and solidity, and can be a liberating experience. We will discuss groundwork versus mounted work in more detail later.

Theory: The deepening stage echoes Bugental's conceptualization of self as being a part of and apart from, as well as the Gestalt concept of the cocreated nature of relationships and sense of self. Within the therapeutic equine community, it is not unusual for individuals to refer to a group of people as a human herd. This reversal of anthropomorphism of ascribing equine qualities to humans may be an indication of the sense of belonging that humans feel when in the company of horses, and is consistent with the idea that when in the company of humans, horses transcend the species barrier and transfer their herd-based relational instincts to people and include them as part of their herd, and thus elicit feelings of belonging. Through the acceptance and non-judgmental nature of the horses, this deepening stage also provides the opportunity for addressing attachment patterns, as the formation of secure attachment is dependent on the caregiver's ability to provide a solid foundation for one's sense of self.

Philosophically, the deepening stage is reminiscent of Merleau-Ponty's view of the living body acting as a mediator between subjectivity and the world, and where the embodied experience connects with the world through intentionality as an active agent in its environment. It is also evocative of Buber's notion that mutual relating between *I-Thou* manifests through the "bodying forth" of the self. Within Gestalt theory, this can be linked to Ruella Frank's concept of the embodied movement of yielding into support as a way to feel more present and grounded within oneself.

STAGE FOUR: COMING HOME

The fourth stage of the HERD Model is a process of embodied reoccupation, and an unfolding to deeper authenticity, and greater intentionality in the present moment. This moment-by-moment unfolding allows clients to let go of expectations and be open to the unexpected, and move toward reclaiming oneself fully in the whole of one's being, both bodily and emotionally. This may involve a heightened awareness of how they curtail their own desires and instincts, allowing them to see more clearly the part they play in any physiological and psychological constriction, and how that impacts the quality of connection with those around them. When we become conscious of what it is we do to distance ourselves from others, and how this blocks contact and connection, we are more able to accept responsibility for our actions.

From my research, participants emphasized the importance of paying greater attention to their own body process as a way of accessing a stronger sense of self-agency. In other words, when they became aware of their embodied presence and movements, they were able to gain a deeper understanding of their way of being in the world and take more responsibility for their own actions. This shift in their sense of self then impacted their way of being with others in relationship, and allowed them to feel a greater sense of belonging to the world around them, and within their relationships. This stage of the process is the journey of returning to a familiar place, and a coming home to self and relationship.

Within the HERD Model, clients are often invited to attend to their immediate awareness of their surroundings and their bodily process in the moment. This may be achieved through a phenomenological exercise in observing themselves in their interactions with the horses, paying attention to what is happening in each moment, catching the stories that they are telling themselves and/or noticing when they are drifting away from the immediate interaction with the horses. This allows the client to give space to what is emerging for them emotionally, physically, and cognitively in the here-and-now, and offers the potential for the reoccupation of their whole being, and the experience of returning to home base as they connect with self, other, and environment.

Theory: From a theoretical lens, this process can be seen as an awakening of the client's latent potential from which they may actualize. This awareness is met with the clients' reclaiming of their own agency and the movement toward a more graceful unfolding of their full potential. This process of embodiment reiterates Merleau-Ponty's concept that "by remaking contact with the body and with the world, we shall also rediscover ourself" as intentional beings. It also corresponds to the core Gestalt tenet of the importance of present moment awareness, and that it is only through paying attention to the here-and-now that we can access a felt-sense of ourselves, which takes into account the fullness of our experience of ourselves to allow for authenticity to emerge.

This is a move away from a habitual process of being in the there-and-then, which takes our awareness to what might happen in the future or what has occurred in the past. The anchoring of awareness in the here-and-now is a process of re-inhabitation in order to experience our bodies, and therefore, our self fully. In this context, the client's embodied experience of the horses and their environment also shifts their embodied sense of themselves. This is the experience of coming home to self and relationship.

STAGE FIVE: INTEGRATION

The final stage of the HERD Model is that of integration. The progression through the five stages culminates in the gathering of all our newfound awareness of self, other, and environment, allowing for an all encompassing and enduring experience. When we experience something new and profound, whether it is a deeper understanding of ourselves, something that moves, motivates, or inspires us, the emotions stirred within may dissipate over time if there is no integration. This final stage is crucial for clients to be able to hold on to their experiences in order for them to translate them into their everyday lives. It is here that we can consolidate new learning to provide an anchor, or home base, for our clients to return to. By supporting clients to mindfully recall their experiences on an embodied level, so that they can feel into that space within themselves while still being in relationship with the therapist and horses, allows them to fully integrate their experience.

Within the HERD Model, clients are encouraged to deepen their sense of being in the moment in order to allow the experience to sink in and become integrated within. This embodied integration is often followed by an exhale or sigh as an indication of an embodied readiness to move onto the next figure, against the backdrop of their ground, lending to a sense of an all encompassing and enduring experience. Through tracking the client's bodily process, the therapist watches for the outbreath as a sign of experiential integration. Toward the end of a session, clients may also be invited to describe in as much detail as possible the feelings, sensations, and movements that have been elicited by their equine encounters. This phenomenological description of what and how the encounter took place, accentuates the embodied impact of their experiences in the here and now. By sinking even deeper into the experience in that moment, clients can solidify their embodied experiences, make meaning from them for themselves, and thereby hold on to the embodied learning from the session. This supports their ability to recall the experience outside of the therapeutic space, and acts as a home base for them to return to at any moment in time. This is an empowering process for many clients who may otherwise struggle to integrate their experiences into their daily lives. This is the fully embodied awareness of self, other, and environment that the HERD Model facilitates.

From my research, participants drew particular attention to their ability to recall their embodied experiential learning, months and even years after the event. This enduring nature of the experience underlines how deeply ingrained the experience had become, and was felt throughout the whole of their being. Full integration occurs when clients are able to feel a sense of timelessness in their ability to recall the event, so that it becomes a constant echo through their bodily being that honors their authentic existence. The enduring nature of full integration allows for clients to bring to surface the same feelings, sensations, and the meanings they made of them when they recall their experiences.

Theory: The Gestalt use of the term "embodied" takes into account the fullness of our experience of our self, internally and externally, in relation to our environment and acknowledges that our body *is* our self. The client's embodied experience pertaining to a sense of timelessness can be viewed as part of the enduring nature of our sense of self within our body; that as long as we exist, our embodied experience remains alive. So in returning to ourselves, to experience ourselves, in this embodied way allows for the experiential learning to become a part of us. As Peter Levine asserts, it is here that "mind and body, thought and feeling, psyche and spirit, are held together, welded in an undifferentiated unity of experience."

SUMMARY

The HERD Model of EFP begins with connecting with the horse through physical touch and shared breath. This intentional act of **sharing space** with another offers the opportunity for further connection. It is often a nonverbal act that acknowledges the step toward being in relation with the horse as another living, sentient being. The experience of being in relationship with a non-human other allows for the **release** from internalized constraints. This may be experienced as a move away from the client's habitually defended ways of encountering others, offering a moment's pause to relax long held restrictions. This release acts as a path toward relationship with another that incorporates an **expansion** that widens the horizons of clients' perspectives of themselves and reveals more of what was previously kept hidden from others. This incorporates taking the risk toward authenticity, and thereby **deepening** their connection and relationships with others. This deepening allows clients to return to a familiar place of belonging where one is recognized by self and other. This process of **coming home** to one's authentic being is a strengthening process of finding solidity in oneself while in relation to another. It is the moment-to-moment unfolding of the fullness of one's bodily and emotional existence, and an **integration** of their experiences. This integration leads to an all encompassing and enduring process through the whole of one's bodily being and is held with a sense of timelessness.

Chapter 8

The HERD Model of Equine Facilitated Learning

The HERD Model of EFL is a synthesis of the philosophical and theoretical principles of the HERD EFP Model, and my experience as a corporate trainer, consultant, and educator. While the underlying principles are the same as those within the EFP model, working in an educational, coaching, or corporate training setting falls within an entirely different scope of practice. This chapter will discuss the boundaries that practitioners need to be aware of within their scope of practice, before introducing the HERD Model of EFL.

SCOPE OF PRACTICE

EFL practitioners are educators, organizational consultants, corporate trainers, human resource professionals, and life coaches who incorporate horses into their work with clients.

Clients may range from high-level executives for Fortune 500 companies, small business owners, adults, and children with special needs, to individuals looking for coaching but not therapy. Clients may be interested in leadership training, team building, assertiveness, conflict resolution, or communication skills. They may want to introduce horses as an educational experience to students with cognitive or emotional challenges as a way to explore social communication skills. They may want to learn about their own management style or need coaching through a particular aspect of their lives. Whatever the presenting goal is, the EFL practitioner needs to understand the context within which their clients operate, and work within safe and ethical boundaries.

EFL clients are NOT attending the session for in-depth personal explorations. The conditions and parameters within the session may not be a safe enough container for them to express themselves fully. Practitioners need to be mindful of this and take care not to leave clients feeling emotionally exposed and unsupported in a group setting. This is not to say that clients cannot be challenged to reflect on their process, but it is important to know where to draw the line. It is imperative that practitioners understand that this is a matter of consent: EFL clients have not signed an informed consent agreement. They have not given consent to be put under the microscope in the same way as a therapy client. Furthermore, without the training and

Equine-Facilitated Psychotherapy and Learning. DOI: http://dx.doi.org/10.1016/B978-0-12-812601-1.00008-0

licensure of a mental health practitioner, it is unethical and outside the scope of practice to offer psychotherapy or counseling interventions. Whilst the interaction with the horses may be therapeutic, this is not therapy. As an EFL practitioner, the aim is to provide learning experiences for clients that are concrete and translatable into everyday life.

Ilka Parent, a leading EFPL practitioner offers a good rule of thumb to follow, and suggests that practitioners ask themselves the question, "If horses were not involved in this interaction, would I still feel competent and qualified to continue with this intervention with this client?" If not, then she suggests that a different course of action is required. This does not mean that clients cannot offer personal insights and information themselves, nor does it mean that this is inappropriate. The important distinction is that it is something they are offering freely, not as a result of an intervention or question that they feel they must answer.

The issue of scope of practice is an important one not only to ensure safe and ethical practice, but an understanding of these parameters also helps practitioners to embody the philosophical and theoretical foundations of the HERD Model. As discussed previously, there is a danger in assuming that if we are to be authentic, we must lay ourselves bare with all our vulnerabilities. Modeling authenticity with boundaries for our EFL clients is perhaps one of the most powerful ways of connecting with them.

THE HERD MODEL OF EFL

This section outlines the HERD Model of EFL as a three-stage process of: Meeting, Relating, and Integrating. Maintaining our philosophical and theoretical foundations, we will explore what it means to lead individual coaching sessions, and corporate or educational groups in an embodied and relational way; and how this impacts the way that clients can begin to relate differently to their colleagues/friends within the group, and in their lives. This approach highlights the importance of practitioner authenticity, as a model for participants to engage with each other through an embodied and authentic self.

Whilst these three stages have clear overlaps with the HERD EFP Model outlined in the previous chapter, there are also significant differences by virtue of the shift in scope of practice.

In particular, the shift in scope of practice leads to differences in the use of reflective language and questioning. Rather than focusing on one person's inner process as it is revealed through their way of relating to the horse(s), the focus is on group process and the intended learning outcomes of the session. This necessitates a pragmatic approach that incorporates the participant's experience in the here-and-now of the session, as well as the wider aims and objectives of the client, who may or may not be in attendance (e.g., the Human Resources Director who sends an accounting team for some team building training).

Stage One: Meeting

The first stage of the HERD Model of EFL is the process of Meeting. By this, I am referring to the process of meeting your clients in a way that honors their situation, regardless of the setup of the facility, client population, and expected outcomes of the session. It also refers to how to introduce your participants to the horses they will be working with. This first stage might begin months, or weeks, before the session itself, and may occur online, via the telephone, or in person. This process begins with your first contact with the client, and includes how you prepare for the session. Meeting, in this sense, is making contact.

Although the HERD Model of EFL is still centered on a relational process, considerations must be given to the client's goals for engaging in the session. "Client" in this setting, refers to the organization/individual contracting your services rather than those participating in the event. Many EFL sessions are either one-time events, or a short series of workshops. Sometimes, the same participants will return for a continuous learning program (such as a 6 week program for elementary school students learning about social interactions), and other times it will be on a rotational basis to allow for everyone within an organizational group to take part in the experience (such as providing the same educational day out for a cancer unit over a number of visits).

Whereas an EFP session follows the client's process as figures emerge, EFL practitioners may already have a preset goal given by clients for the corporate team, psychosocial, or psycho-educational class in attendance. For example, for an organizational team-building event, the participants arrive with the mindset of working on team dynamics and the session will be preframed on this basis. For this reason, it is important to have a sense of the context of the participants before their arrival. For this, the HERD Model recommends a thorough need analysis with the main contact for the event in order to design and deliver a session with the most impact.

Meeting a Need

In order to design a program that meets the needs of participants coming to an EFL program, we must first distinguish between the different client groups that we may encounter.

1. **Task based:** The purpose of these groups is to enhance the overall function of the group in relation to specific goals and outcomes. For example, team communication, leadership, or conflict resolution in organizations.
2. **Psychosocial:** The purpose of these groups is to provide learning to enhance social functioning of individuals within the group. For example, working with Alzheimer's patients from a nursing home to engage them in grooming and petting horses.

3. **Psychoeducational:** The purpose of these groups is to provide educational opportunities related to psychological functioning. For example, working with at-risk adolescents through a vocational program that highlights responsibility, boundaries, and teamwork.

The first contact with a client within the EFL setting is often with the organizer of the event, rather than with the participants themselves. The main contact may or may not be in attendance at the actual event. Depending on the set up of the organization the EFL program is operating from, it may fall to the practitioner to occupy a number of roles: Event coordinator, sales and marketing person, administrator, and EFL event trainer/educator/coach. In order meet the needs of the clients, it is important to understand the responsibilities behind each of these roles, and how they support the development, design, and implementation of any training or educational program. When operating as a small business or sole practitioner, these responsibilities may fall on one person, and often becomes a balancing act in order to meet the needs of different clients.

Fig. 8.1 shows the process from first contact with clients through to follow-up postprogram delivery. By the time we reach this cycle, there may already have been a number of meetings and/or conversations with the client to ascertain their needs and to engage them enough to commit to the EFL

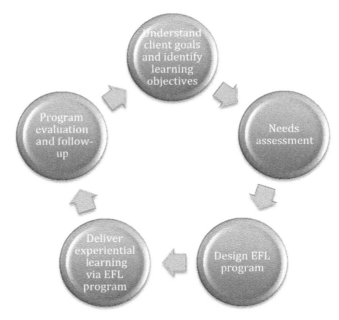

FIGURE 8.1   Training/education implementation cycle.

program. It is strongly advised for the EFL practitioner to have made direct contact with the client contracting your services before delivering any session. The following are important general questions to consider for a practitioner leading up to this and moving through the cycle:

a. Does the client have direct contact with the practitioner running the event? Or are they dealing with an administrator responsible for event coordination? If it is the latter, how does the information gleaned from the initial contact with the client transfer to the lead practitioner? Does the administrator have training and knowledge to be able to ascertain client needs and learning objectives? If not, what is the process of communication and what basic information does he/she need to elicit from the client for the practitioner to be able to build on?

b. What considerations need to be taken into account for the cognitive, emotional, or physical constraints of the participants? Are there any specific health and safety concerns that need to be taken into consideration in the design of the program?

c. What does the client hope for participants to achieve as a result of this program? What specific skill would the client like participants to gain as a result of this program? Is there an action specific learning objective that can be formulated for the event? What is the learning or skill gap that is being addressed by the program? Is this something that is achievable in one session, or would it be better to design a program series? What might the client want/need from the EFL provider in order to commit to a program series?

d. What is the EFL practitioner's experience of the participant population? Does the program reflect the skills and strengths of the EFL delivery team? What activities might be suitable for the learning objectives set? Which horses would be compatible with the activities being considered? Will there be any mounted activities? Are there participants in attendance who may have contraindications for being mounted? What additional staff or volunteer support might be needed if mounted activities are offered?

e. Who is responsible for coordinating the joining instructions and information for attendance? What information will be provided to participants prior to the program delivery? What is the duration of the program? How will the event be managed in terms of registrations, logistics, administration, and staffing (horses and humans), both in the lead up to delivery, on the day, and in follow-up evaluations? How will program evaluations be administered? What amenities are available at the facility, and how will the event be structured to suit the layout of the facility? Indoors? Outdoors? Is there a Plan B for inclement weather?

Meeting the needs of participants during the delivery phase of the program cycle may at first seem like it should take first priority. However, without adequate preparation in the lead up to delivery, and a rigorous evaluation process, it is invariably problematic to meet expectations. Assuming that the ground has been prepared for this, meeting the needs of the participants during the program delivery requires us to meet the participants with openness and willingness to engage with them in their world.

Meeting the Participant

Drawing from our philosophical traditions of an embodied phenomenological way of relating, the HERD Model of EFL places an emphasis on a noninterpretative and descriptive approach to facilitation. Regardless of the design of the EFL session, the role of the practitioner is to facilitate the participant's encounter with the horse(s). Whether we are working with a large or small group, or on an individual basis, it is imperative to maintain a safe container for participants to express and explore their experiences. This means that practitioners need to be mindful of issues of confidentiality and make it explicit that anything that is shared within the group, is not shared outside of it, and that any conversations about a participant's individual experience about what happened during the session, must be kept to reflections about their own process and not about anyone else in the group. This is important when working within any group setting, whether it is an educational, small business, or corporate environment. It is only natural for participants to talk about their experiences with the horses after the event with friends, families, and/or colleagues. In the wider context of school and work, it is important that these experiences do not become fodder for the gossip mill. Making this explicit at the beginning helps participants to feel more at ease with sharing their experiences throughout the session. By demonstrating an understanding of the context within which the participant's lived experiences emerge, the practitioner is able to take the first step towards meeting the participant in their space.

The ability to meet our participants by looking at the world through their eyes is essentially an existential-humanistic perspective that takes into account the phenomenal experience of each individual. It is foundational to the HERD approach and the principles behind experiential learning.

EXPERIENTIAL LEARNING

Carl Rogers, the father of the humanistic approach to psychology, believed that all learning should be student led, and that learners are inspired through the personal integrity of their trainer/teacher. By developing empathy and trust, a trainer/teacher can enable students to realize their true potential and achieve personal growth.

For experiential learning theory, we turn to the model of Kolb's learning cycle. This centers on the idea that people learn through past experiences by a process of reflection, and then consequently trying out new ideas. The learning cycle draws together concepts from behavioral and cognitive schools of thought and is based on the works of Lewin, Dewey, and Piaget, who are seen as leaders in traditional learning psychology.

Kurt Lewin was a Gestalt psychotherapist who believed that individuals rely on concrete experiences to be able to make sense of abstract ideas. Educational reformist and psychologist, John Dewey, explored how learning occurs despite conflicts between concrete experiences of an individual, and the abstract ideas presented, and how these conflicts may be resolved to obtain a higher level of learning. Dewey believed that personal experiences stimulate ideas for learning, and that this is crucial to any learning process. His pragmatic approach centers on learning through doing. Developmental psychologist, Jean Piaget's, contribution towards Kolb's theory focuses on the interaction between the individual and their learning environment. His theories of accommodation and assimilation are clearly evident within the learning cycle, where an individual must accept new ideas and concepts, and interpret them on a cognitive level, in order for learning to occur. This implies that learning is the reconciliation of personal experience and expectations, such that learning is essentially the creation and re-creation of existing knowledge.

Kolb's interpretation of the work of these theorists led him to present the learning cycle as:

1. Concrete experience
2. Observations and reflections
3. Formation of abstract concepts and generalizations
4. Testing implications of concepts in new situations

These stages form a continuous cycle, where learning can begin at any stage and is an ongoing process.

This framework is compatible with the phenomenological and relational approach of the HERD Model of EFL as it positions learning as a holistic process. From this perspective, a holistic and integrative approach to learning that combines experience, perception, cognition, and behavior, allows for experiences to become embedded as learning. Learning, in this sense, incorporates the broadening of psychological awareness, and the gaining of personal insight to one's relational process. Experiential learning naturally becomes one's lived experience, so is therefore also an *embodied* process.

In terms of meeting the participant, the implications of Kolb's learning cycle within coaching, training and educational environments are such that programs should be designed to acknowledge that participants engage in the learning process by bringing their own experiences into the present moment. The role of the HERD practitioner is to facilitate learning while allowing the participant's experiences to act as a backdrop for increased awareness.

From our theoretical foundations, this is consistent with the Gestalt principle of figure/ground. As we meet our participants on their ground, focusing on the figure that emerges, we are more able to be present with them in their lived experience of the here-and-now. In this way, we can invite participants to step into the space we create for learning, and walk alongside them on their journey of self-discovery.

When we regard learning as a socially situated process, it allows us to embrace the interconnectedness between us. When participants feel empowered through their learning, they become more able to participate in their communities, and more likely to establish relationships with others, share their knowledge and its application, thus creating a ripple effect within their communities. This process involves the gradual movement of the individual from peripheral to full participation in their communities, and broadens their horizons, and invites authentic relatedness.

Meeting the Horses

Facilitating participants' first meeting with the horses within an EFL session requires forethought and planning. Regardless of the size of the group and/or individual participant's prior experience with horses (or not), it is imperative that participants are fully briefed on The HERD Safety Protocols before interacting with the horses. Practitioners must also take into account the number of horses they are partnering with, relative to the group size in attendance, and ensure that they have adequate assistance, in the form of equine support staff or adjuvants, on hand to help in keeping both horses and humans safe. The process of meeting the herd is much more structured than that of an EFP session, and the practitioner is required to provide more direction in their style of facilitation.

My experience in leading EFL groups has revealed that preparing to meet the horses is as important as the actual meeting. Practitioners need to be cognizant of the comfort/anxiety level of their participants. For some people, horses are intimidating. For many others, horses are completely unfamiliar. There have been many occasions when participants have expressed their fear and anxiety about being in the proximity of horses due to a childhood accident, or simply being inexperienced with such large animals.

To support this process, we return to our foundations of breath and embodied awareness. During the first session with any group, I often begin with asking everyone to introduce themselves, and to let me know how they feel about spending some time at the barn. Before we go into the barn itself, I will lead them through a grounding exercise to encourage them to get back in touch with their bodily being. Breathing together as a group, and releasing some tensions in our bodies, allows us to free up some space to be open to new encounters. As described in the previous chapter, when we begin to share space with another being in a conscious and intentional way, we are taking a risk to open up.

My preference in conducting any EFL session is to allow participants the opportunity to observe a herd of horses at liberty. Whether this is out in a paddock or in an arena, the experience of watching these majestic animals freely interacting with each other always brings an element of awe. Encouraging participants to pay attention first to their own embodied experiences as they observe the horses, and then to the stories they might be telling themselves about what they are observing, allows participants to ease into this meeting space between self, other, and environment.

To facilitate this process calls upon the practitioner to act as a model for the participants in how to meet each other with presence and authenticity. The practitioner, along with the Equine Support Staff if one is present, is also an advocate for their equine partners, and must take into consideration their needs during any interaction with the participants. In my EFL work, I have found it to be both a humbling and inspiring process to lead participants through the risky terrain of truly meeting the horses and then each other, sometimes for the first time, from a place of embodied authenticity.

STAGE TWO: RELATING

If we are to fully subscribe to a phenomenological and I-Thou relational approach to meeting our participants, then we must first acknowledge the assumption that is often present about working in this way; that is, that there is a right and wrong way of being authentic. What I mean by this is that practitioners need to be mindful of their own assumptions about what "authenticity" looks/feels like to them, and not to position it as a goal for participants to reach for. Consistent with our philosophical foundations, authenticity is not a concrete "thing" that one has or doesn't have. Rather, it is a collection of fleeting moments of connection between self, other, and environment. It is an ever evolving, ebb and flow of intentional and relational focus, and process of being-in-the-world.

The notion of being true to oneself as a concrete mark of authenticity is antithetical to the existential and Gestalt traditions of the HERD approach. Instead, we view participants as a work in progress (and self as process), avoiding any static labeling of the person and behaviors. By staying open and curious to what may emerge for the individual and/or group within the EFL session, we can maintain a phenomenological and I-Thou attitude toward participants, and remain descriptive in our observations of the process between participants and the horses. Thus, participants are not "resistant" or "defensive," and nor are the horses "reactive" or "disruptive." Practitioners can maintain an active curiosity, or in Gestalt terms, "creative indifference" to the process unfolding before them. Creative indifference calls for the practitioner to bracket our own assumptions (i.e., it is part of the phenomenological attitude), and also any agendas that may have emerged; it is the practice of allowing the process to unfold in whatever direction without an invest-ment in the outcome.

This way of relating to both participants and horses allows the practi-tioner the freedom to describe what they are witnessing, and offer the obser-vations back to the participants to draw meaning from within their own context. The art of facilitation in this setting is for practitioners to make keen observations of the interactions between participants and the horses, paying particular attention to the non-verbal elements of interaction, and relating them to the context through reflective questioning. Interventions such as ask-ing the group, "How did the horse respond to your request?" or "What do you notice about how the horses are interacting?" and "What happened when you saw your friends doing this?" encourages the group to express their col-lective, and individual, lived experiences of that moment. The process is not only focused on the metaphorical aspects of what may emerge in the session, but on the actual lived experience of the relationships that are formed in the moment between the horses and the participants.

In holding space for a relational process, it is the practitioner's responsi-bility to facilitate dialogue and interactions between participants and the horses, and step out of the central focus of the process. Redirecting com-ments by asking questions such as "What would you like your team to know?" and "Would anyone like to respond to that?" or "Who else resonates with that?" rather than the practitioner responding to each participant, allows the process to unfold within the group in an organic manner. By fostering the idea that participants can learn from the horses and from each other, and not only from the practitioner, provides a more inclusive and level playing field for learning. Through engaging with participants as equals rather than as expert, we allow space for participants to step forward and connect with each other in their own way.

STAGE THREE: INTEGRATING

The purpose of any EFL session is for participants to return to their daily lives with an experience that is translatable to their context. This may be learning how to make friends at elementary school, or decreasing negative behaviors for Alzheimer's patients, or increasing focus for autistic children, or working more cohesively within a team. Whatever the client population, the process of integration begins during the EFL session.

I want you to think about a training or educational event that you attended that moved or changed you in a profound way. Remember what you felt in your body; the sensations and emotions, and try and pinpoint the moment that you began to notice that feeling. Remember the shift in your embodied consciousness that alerted you to the seed that was sown. It may have been so subtle and almost imperceptible in the beginning but grew into something that you couldn't ignore. It may have felt like a lightning bolt that is shockingly seared into your memory. Perhaps it was a smoldering fire that refused to be extinguished. Maybe it felt like the uncomplicated, undemanding, and patient unearthing of the parts of you that had been deeply buried. Take yourself back to that time and place where you felt deeply impacted by a new experience.

What you experienced in that moment is what I refer to as the **MAGIC** of learning integration. The elements that make up a successful coaching, training, or educational experience that leads to learning that sticks:

Memorable
Applicable
Generous
Inspiring
Creative

The experience must be **memorable** in a way that excites and energizes participants when they recall the event to others. It must be **applicable** to their daily lives and fit within their situational context, so that the lessons learned can become attached to real life scenarios. Participants must feel **generous** about sharing the ideas that they have learned and telling others about their experience. This fosters an **inspiring** environment for others around them to want to gain a similar experience, and to share in the learning. Finally, the learning must lead to a **creative** process of integration for the participant, where he/she can envision a different way of being-in-the world as a result of the experience.

These elements directly correspond with feedback provided following the coaching/training/educational sessions provided by The HERD Institute. Participants said that as they recalled the details of the event, they were able to feel the same sensations in their bodies as they did in the moment, and remember the lessons that they took from the experience. Participants also stated that they talked about their experience to friends and family, long after the event, and encouraged colleagues to attend a session if given the opportunity. Participants were also creative in the ways that they utilized their learning, and stated that they would return to the themes that emerged from the session, and refer to this collectively within their class or team as a way of cementing the new insights gained as a result of the experience.

THEMES, CULTURE, AND LANGUAGE

Due to the diverse client population that EFL sessions cover, it is important for practitioners to develop an adaptable facilitation style that is appropriate for the participants. Running an EFL session for an elementary school group on respecting personal boundaries is very different to facilitating a conflict resolution session for a corporate team. However, the exercises and the principles behind the sessions may be the same. The art of facilitation is in listening deeply to the themes that emerge from the participants themselves, and tracking the progress of the development of the theme throughout the session. Within any organizational team or educational group, there will be a microculture of norms and implicitly shared values, beliefs, and rituals. In order to engage the group, the practitioner needs to be aware of some these elements of the group culture and adapt quickly to the shared language and ways of being within it. This is what the horses are particularly skilled at facilitating.

When we focus on the embodied relational process between the participants and the horses, we are able to connect on a deeper level to the way in which participants are bringing themselves into relationship with each other. This, in turn, provides immediate feedback to them as to how they may be received by others within their team or group. The integration of learning occurs at a deeper level as a result of this embodied process and lived experience. For some client populations, such as non-verbal autistic individuals attending an EFL session on enhancing social skills, the embodied experiential learning removes the need to focus on cognitive processing.

As discussed previously, since the embodied experience is so ineffable, the language used by practitioners during an EFL session needs to be considered with the utmost care, and is highly dependent on the client population you are working with. For each specific client group, it is useful to gain an understanding of any specific jargon as reference points for linking to themes that may emerge during the session. In this way, we can step into the world of our participants and walk with them for a while.

SUMMARY

The HERD Model of EFL is founded on the same philosophical and theoretical principles as the HERD EFP model. Maintaining a phenomenological and I-Thou relational approach to meeting participants in their space, the focus is placed on the relationships built between participants and the horses. While learning objectives may be set prior to the event by the clients, the format of an EFL session still holds space for the immediacy of the moment for collective themes to emerge. Practitioners working within the HERD EFL Model must ensure that they are proficient in their ability to maintain the boundaries within their scope of practice, and pay attention to issues of confidentiality and emotional safety of participants during a session. The use of reflective and inclusive language allows for participants to ponder their responses to what is happening in the here-and-now, and provides a welcoming space for them to share their experiences.

The HERD EFL Model is a three-stage process:

MEETING: Clients, Participants & Horses

RELATING: Phenomenological, Reflective & Inclusive

INTEGRATING: MAGIC of Learning

It incorporates the considerations necessary for **meeting** the needs of clients, participants, and horses. The aim is to foster a learning environment that is supportive of an embodied process of **relating** for participants. This is a phenomenological process of inquiry that emphasizes the use of reflective and inclusive language and questions by the practitioner. This, in turn, provides the conditions necessary for **integrating** through the MAGIC of learning. These elements are supported throughout by the practitioner's awareness and development of the themes, culture, and language that is applicable to the client population being served. At the heart of the HERD EFL Model, is the belief that all learning is an interconnected, holistic, and embodied process.

Chapter 9

The HERD Model of EFP in Action

When I'm asked about my work with horses, I am often met with a puzzled look and a dose of skepticism. Although equine therapy as an umbrella term is becoming more mainstream, and it is gaining some exposure through media coverage, it is more often associated with therapeutic riding rather than mental health programs. Both the general public and medical practitioners are under-informed as to what EFP is, and it therefore appears to lack legitimacy. Criticisms also abound about the lack of empirical research available in the field of EFP in general, let alone any specific modality. Additionally, due to the differing approaches under the umbrella of EFPL, meta-analyses of treatment programs do not provide like-for-like comparisons. The studies that have been peer-reviewed and published are often qualitative and not quantitative, and therefore seen as undeserving of attention and/or validity. While I recognize that there is merit in quantitative research, and that it is needed in our field, I also want to emphasize that qualitative research is not to be dismissed.

At the HERD Institute, we believe that research is a priority and promote the importance of research as a way to increase the credibility of EFPL. We also strongly believe that a phenomenological and qualitative research methodology is a natural fit for the HERD model of EFPL. Particularly given the philosophical and theoretical foundations of the HERD approach, a qualitative research method allows for a true reflection of the work being examined. Moreover, while quantitative studies maybe somewhat useful in assessing treatment efficacy, they do not provide the reader with a sense of what the work looks and feels like in action. This section aims to provide the reader with a textured description of the work in action. It includes some of my personal reflections, interactions, and learning from my own experiences as well as case studies of clients I have worked with.

Over the years, I have had the privilege of working with many different herds across the States and in the United Kingdom. These case studies shine a light on these horses and the incredible healing they have facilitated. They come from a diverse background, including those rescued from slaughter, supporting students at a therapeutic riding facility, those exclusively working as EFPL partners, regular riding lesson mounts, retired schoolmasters, off the

Equine-Facilitated Psychotherapy and Learning. DOI: http://dx.doi.org/10.1016/B978-0-12-812601-1.00009-2

track thoroughbreds, retired Amish work horses, and of course, my own herd of horses at The HERD Institute. Each of the horses mentioned in this chapter, and the next, have willingly and generously opened their hearts to my clients, demonstrating their unwavering support and solid presence. I have been humbled by their wisdom, strength, and resilience, and it is with heartfelt gratitude and a continued sense of awe that I share these journeys with our clients, and some personal reflections with you.

YOU HAD ME AT HELLO

I have a habit of picking horses that my trainers think are "unsuitable" for me. First, there was Rupert, the Goth-Rock pony that stole my heart the instant I met him. He was barreling around the arena, black mane flying, tail flicking, and head tossing, clearly disgruntled at his rider for daring to ask him to lower his head and collect his stride. When he came sliding to a halt in front of me, he stuck his muzzle in my hair and sneezed. I was smitten.

Rupert was a jet black Fell Pony, solidly built, and only 5 years old at the time. He had been trained as a driving pony, and was about as inexperienced as I was, so it was understandable that my trainer had reservations when I insisted that I wanted to work with him.

I worked with Rupert for about 3 years, leasing him after about 6 months of meeting him. He taught me so much, not only in terms of horsemanship, but also about forgiveness. I would fall off, get back on, rinse, and repeat. Each time I fell, he would realize I had disembarked, and slowly walk back over to me as I lay on the ground, lower his muzzle, and breathe on my head. I was not aware at that point what it was that kept drawing me back into the relationship, but this simple gesture touched my heart, and despite my trainer's concerns, my gut told me to hang in there with him.

As it turned out, about a year into our relationship, there were times when I couldn't ride due to medical reasons. Instead, I spent time watching him in his paddock while he was out grazing, mesmerized by his antics with his herd. He was a playful boy and full of energy, so it was not unusual for him to gallop around the field bucking and kicking to get attention from his pasture mates. When I entered into his space, he would come and greet me in his usual way by sticking his muzzle on my head and breathing on me. I would walk around the pasture with him following me, and when I needed to rest, I would sit under a tree, and he would stand or lie down next to me. I treasured those moments of connection, and it changed my relationship with horses into one of being with rather than doing to.

My experience with Rupert gave me a taste of the joy and depth of love and connection that was possible between horse and human. I grieved the loss of him for a long time when we moved to the United States. It took me a while to even begin to want to connect with another horse. When I eventually started to think about leasing another horse, I realized that I couldn't go through that process again, so I decided to take the leap and buy one of my own.

Reba was the 25th horse I went to see. That's how careful I was about picking the right partner. I wanted a horse that was quiet, soft, and gentle, who would be open to connecting with me and with whom I could partner with in my equine-facilitated therapy work. I wanted a horse that was steady enough to withstand that unpredictable nature of clients with cognitive, emotional, and physical challenges so that I could build on my therapeutic riding instructor experience. I wanted a horse that I could take on trail rides and just hang out with. Most of all, I wanted a horse that would enjoy doing all those things with me.

My first glimpse of Reba was of her standing quietly, cross-tied in the barn aisle. As I walked up to her, she looked at me and dropped her head onto my shoulder. I stroked her, patted her, lifted up her feet, and she welcomed me into her space with a soft and gentle eye. I was hooked.

My trainers were shocked at my choice in Reba. While they had been advising me to buy a been there done that, broke and finished, gelding to fit with the hunter/jumper and dressage environment I was used to, I chose a broodmare with a reining and cutting pedigree, who had never seen a jump. On paper, Reba was completely "unsuitable" for me, and yet I experienced the same sensation as I had with Rupert. I felt my body soften, relax, and open up toward her. There was no question in my heart that she was the one. Over the years, others have tried to persuade me otherwise, and I came close to believing them. And yet, as with Rupert, I listened to my instincts and stuck with her. I now understand our journey to be one of trust: in myself, in her, and in relationships.

So often, we are taught to value evidence-based, statistical, rational, and logical analyses over innate sensations, emotions, and inner wisdom. Whether we are working with corporate teams or individuals, couples, or families in therapy, placing an emphasis on the need to search for answers outside of themselves, would neglect our clients' own sense of value and intrinsic knowledge as well as their felt experiences. From an existential-humanistic perspective, it is precisely these felt experiences that we focus on in order to illuminate what has been kept hidden from the world and ourselves. Our aim is to support the embodiment of our authentic way of being in the world that allows us to expand our horizons. Sometimes, the noise that surrounds us makes it hard to listen to our own truth; other voices of authority, and echoes from the past, clamor for attention to dilute the message from within. That is not to say there is no place in the world for evidence-based and scientific knowledge, but it is not the only way.

Challenging our philosophical foundations by asking, "How do we know what we know?" and "How does that impact on how we interact with each other?" is an integral part of the process in any relationship. This is how we release long held restrictions or beliefs, and expand into authenticity; and it is how we facilitate the meeting of our hearts and minds.

Listening deeply to the emotions that Rupert and Reba stirred up within me allowed me to recognize my embodied experience of being seen by another. Sometimes, it's like a lightning bolt that shocks and brightens up the dark sky. Sometimes, it's a smoldering fire that refuses to be extinguished. Often, it is felt as the uncomplicated, undemanding, and patient unearthing of the parts of us that have been deeply buried. When experienced repeatedly over time, this feeling alerts us that we are in the presence of authenticity, and we name it Love. This does not mean that the relationship is smooth and without challenges. It means a commitment to staying in relationship with the other, and willingness to work through the sticky parts, while holding space for the other's truth to emerge. It allows us to trust ourselves, our instincts, and felt sense to find meaning in our lives for ourselves.

This is the type of space we aim to hold for our members at The HERD Institute. We believe wholeheartedly in the potential for individuals to be their own leader, and to forge their own paths toward whatever fulfillment or success means to them. So turn down the noise. Which path feels right for you? What does your heart say? Feel it, believe it, trust it, and allow us to journey with you.

NEW BEGINNINGS: TAKING THE FIRST STEP

I've lived in many places throughout my life; different countries, cities, and towns, and each time I move, I learn something about the way I orient myself in order to find my feet. My last move, in 2013, was particularly difficult. After a wonderful 2 years in Northern Virginia working as an equine-facilitated therapist specializing in eating disorders, I had to close my practice and pass it over to a trusted colleague and start again in a different state. Being told by well-meaning friends and family that "When one door closes, another one opens," left me feeling unsupported in my need to grieve. It was a new beginning that was also a painful ending.

I missed my friends and colleagues, and the herd of horses I worked with. I missed the community that I had become a part of. I missed the diversity of Northern Virginia, and I missed the woodlands where I walked with my dog. I noticed that as I tried to settle into my new life, I compared everything with what had been lost. While I was excited to begin a new journey in Ohio, I also recognized that I wasn't ready to let go and step forward wholeheartedly into it.

I was fortunate enough to be able to bring my mare, Reba, with me to Ohio, so was able to watch her transition into her new life as I eased myself into mine. Since then, she has moved three more times to different facilities. I learnt a lot from observing how she interacted with her new herds, and subsequently have been able to translate that into my own process.

Like us, horses remember their friends, so I have often wondered how they deal with herd transitions. Whether it is pasture mates leaving or if they are the ones that leave, I wonder if they miss their friends and how they feel about entering a new herd. Unlike us, they often don't have a choice as to where they live, or with whom they share their lives, and I wonder what that's like for them.

Watching Reba meeting and greeting a new herd is fascinating to me. I am in awe of what I perceive as her ability to get her bearings of where she has arrived with such ease. Entering into the herd, she is inevitably greeted by other members in turn, during which she will perform her little ritual of sniff, stamp, and squeal. I have yet to see her meet another horse without this little dance of announcing her arrival. I see it as her willingness to engage with others while setting clear boundaries right from the start. Once the dance is over, Reba always chooses to spend time by herself away from the rest of her new herd. Regardless of whether it is a large herd or a small one, a mixed herd or mares only, she will take herself off away from the others to graze by herself for a while. If other horses approach her, she will greet them cautiously and wait to see if they are demanding anything of her. If not, she will return to grazing and allow them into her space. If the other horses are approaching to claim their own space, she will move aside and find another spot for herself. In this way, within a day or so, Reba will find a pasture mate or two to graze alongside. These will become the horses that she stays loyal to during her time in that herd. They will be the ones who she greets vocally when they return to the paddock after being ridden by their owners, and they will be the ones she calls to when she walks by their stalls when I lead her through the barn.

Watching Reba, I became more aware of my own need to allow myself to take some time in surveying my new surroundings, and to assess with whom I wanted to spend time with. I recognized that I needed to find my own human "herd" in order to feel connected with where I had landed, and acknowledged that taking the first step toward that was not easy. It requires taking a risk to show our vulnerabilities and willingness to be open to new relationships.

We are wired for connection and belonging. When we are removed from the safety of our "herd," our brains are literally searching to replace that which was lost. Stepping into a new space is anxiety provoking for many, and we deal with that anxiety in many ways: overcompensate by being extra gregarious, shrink and retreat into the safety of ourselves, or take tentative steps forward and back until we feel secure enough to reveal more of ourselves to those around us.

The beauty of being with horses is that they help us call attention to where we are in our process. I don't know if Reba misses her old pasture mates from previous barns, but I do know that she is able to be present with her current ones in the present moment. Reba reminds me with every move that it is imperative to remain authentic in what we are searching for: connection with others who allow us to be ourselves. It's the type of connection where it is felt on an embodied level as the gradual easing of physical tension, as an opening outward to receive the beauty of friendship. It is the feeling of embracing all of oneself that may often be kept small in everyday life. It is the sensation of not needing to hide, and instead breathe in and be, however we are in each moment, and know that we will be granted deep affective reciprocity. It is the feeling of coming home to a place where one wants to linger and stay awhile.

This is the foundational philosophy of sharing space at The HERD Institute that we foster. The inclusion and acceptance of members as they are in each moment, witnessed and strengthened by the presence of the horse and human herd. We recognize that taking that first step is a difficult one, so we take care to create a safe and nurturing space. We also know that taking that first step toward joining the HERD is the new beginning in a journey of self-discovery, and encourage each new herd member to savor each moment.

CASE STUDIES

This chapter aims to immerse you in the lives of a diverse range of clients I have worked with over the years. Their personal details have been altered to preserve their anonymity and confidentiality, but the essence of their journeys remains intact. The first four case studies are discussed in terms of the HERD model of EFP to clearly illustrate the clinical application of the philosophical and theoretical foundations of this approach. This is followed by a number of case studies demonstrating the wide-ranging clinical application of the HERD model of EFP.

CASE STUDY 1: AMY'S STORY

Sharing Space

The day before Amy's first session with me was traumatic. I had only just started working at the therapeutic equine facility the week before, and was partnering with an outpatient eating disorders clinic that had started referring clients to me there. The night before our first session, three horses in the herd were randomly attacked. A teenage boy had slashed the horses with a machete leaving deep gashes across their hindquarters. Thankfully, the injuries were not fatal and the veterinarian was able to attend to the wounds and administer some painkillers. Less than 24 hours after the attack, the horses were back in their paddock grazing, while the human staff members were still reeling in shock.

Amy had been referred to me by the clinic, newly released from her latest stint in residential care for the treatment of anorexia nervosa. At 16 years old, Amy had already been battling this disorder for 4 years, had been in and out of residential care, and was severely depressed and actively self-harming. Her primary therapist at the clinic had been working with her for 2 years and thought that an equine-facilitated approach might ease her jaded attitude toward traditional office-based therapies. Amy had been exposed to cognitive-behavioral, dialectical-behavioral, psychodrama, art, and nutritional therapies, in individual, group, and family settings. Nothing seemed to break through enough for her to be able to sustain her recovery. From an existential-humanistic approach, my focus in working with Amy was to introduce her to a more experiential process in an attempt to connect with her on an embodied level.

Amy arrived at her first session with me dressed in a baggy long-sleeved sweatshirt that was at least two sizes too big for her. She stuck her hands through the sleeves of the opposite arms of her sweatshirt, and hugged her-self tightly as she stood with her head tilted toward the ground, avoiding any eye contact. Her long, greasy hair hung over her face as she rocked back and forth on her heels.

Looking at Amy, I noticed that I was holding my breath, so intentionally took a couple of deep, audible breaths to center myself. I asked her to pay attention to her own breathing and invited her to join me in taking some deep breaths together before heading into the paddock to meet the horses. Amy obliged by taking a few short, shallow sips of air that she barely let out through her exhale.

As we walked into the paddock where the horses were grazing, I noticed her pulling at the ends of her sleeves. Her eyes were downcast and her breathing was still shallow, but she fixed a smile on her face in answer to every question I asked. The horses were at the opposite end of the paddock, about a hundred feet away from where we stood, when she noticed their inju-ries. I told her what had happened the day before as she stood rooted to the spot, transfixed by their scars, but still continuing to pull her sleeves down over her hands.

> Me: I notice how you're pulling your sleeves over your hands
> Amy: Yeah, it's a bad habit I have. I feel self-conscious of my scars.

Amy pauses and squints at the horses still grazing in the distance; I wait to see what meaning she is making from seeing their scars.

> Me: What do you see?
> Amy: They don't seem to care about their scars. They don't seem to be paying any attention to us either.
> Me: No, they don't seem to. Would you like to get their attention?

Amy ponders for a moment before taking a couple of steps toward the horses and stops.

> Amy: I don't want to force them to be friends with me, but I do want them to notice that I'm here.
> Me: How would you like to get them to notice you?

Amy begins to roll her sleeves up and slowly extends her arms, palms facing upward, toward the horses. As she does this, the three injured horses raised their heads, stopped grazing, and began to move towards us. The rest of the herd remained at a distance and continued to graze. Amy stood still with her arms outreached, with her scars on display on her forearms, as one by one the horses came towards her. They took it in turn to slowly sniff her arms before moving over to make space for the next horse to do the same. When all three horses had greeted her, they remained standing around her, waiting attentively. Amy breathed deeply, slowly exhaled, and began to cry softly. As she cried, one of the horses, Spirit, stepped forward, rested her head on Amy's shoulder, and breathed out. Throwing her arms around the horse, Amy began to sob. As she cried, the horse leaned into her, and I encouraged Amy to lean in and feel the embodied sensation of the horse supporting her full weight. I paid attention to her breathing, and raised her awareness to it by encouraging her to breathe in synch with the horse. As she began to slow her breathing, she started to stroke Spirit with each exhale. One breath, one movement. Throughout this encounter, the other two injured horses remained by her side. This moment-by-moment unfolding of the beginnings of how Amy made contact with the horses sparked an exploration of what it meant for her to share space with another in relationships.

This first stage of the HERD model of EFP of **sharing space** can clearly be seen in action in Amy's interactions with the horses. This intentionally relational act of breathing and movement allowed Amy to access her own embodied experience. Entering into the herd, in this example, became a mutual encounter that began at a distance before gently moving into a more intimate space. This experience of sharing space supported Amy to breathe more fully, activating her parasympathetic nervous system and calm the body. By staying with a descriptive and phenomenological stance in my observations of her interactions, Amy was able to make meaning of the encounter for herself.

RELEASE AND EXPAND

Amy explained that she spends most of her time trying to hide her scars, her pain, and her eating disorder, not just to everyone else around her, but also to herself; that this process, in her words, "is eating [her] up inside"; and every time she feels that she might have made a connection with someone, that person ends up leaving because her anorexia is too much for him/her to bear witness to. Amy longed to "just be herself" with people. The horses had accepted her without question and stayed with her in her pain. This embodied experience of support and acceptance allowed her to recognize how she abandons her own existence through self-harming and anorexic behaviors, and was something that we returned to as we continued to work together.

Anorexia nervosa can be conceptualized as the ultimate in existential inauthenticity, where the constraints on being are so rigid that it results in the starving of oneself of existence itself, perhaps in an effort to mask the terror of being more visible in the world. In this process, I am often faced with witnessing a slow and deliberate extinction of life and the welcome of bodily death. Questions which may arise in this process include: What aspect of his/her life does the client want to end; what makes living an impossible choice; and what does it feel like on an embodied level to be conflicted about living or dying? These questions may invoke the actuality of experiences for clients who have become numb to their destructive process, or they may act as metaphors for clients to rest their experiences on. There is a paradox within this dilemma in the client's own feelings of worthlessness that drives them toward thinness, believing that once thinness is achieved, he or she would be worthy to live, love, and survive. Yet, it is in the client's striving for that same thinness that will potentially cause death.

Amy's journey continued with a focus on her felt sense of being "too much" for those around her. She was literally making herself smaller in order to confront this existential fear. This smallness can be conceptualized through Kirk Schnieder's constrictive/expansive continuum, where Amy constricted not just her fear, but all sensations of living. Over several months, we worked with the horses by being on the ground and on horseback as she began to reoccupy her sense of herself. This approach included experimenting with mindfully grooming the horse while paying attention to her breathing; leading the horse around the arena while focusing on her physical sense of boundaries; energetically connecting to a horse at liberty, resulting in the horse following her every move around the arena; and lying bareback, spine to spine with the horse, and feeling herself being fully supported. This last experiment was exceptionally challenging for Amy, as it required her to trust that she was not too heavy a burden for me, or her horse, to carry, both literally and figuratively.

In this session, she had chosen to work with one of the smaller horses, Spirit, who also happened to be the one who had initially supported her crying in the first session. We had spent some time grooming and preparing for a bareback mounted session in the indoor arena. Once Spirit had her bareback pad in place, I asked Amy if she felt ready to mount. In order to mount bareback, riders may need a "leg up" even with a mounting block in place. I explained that I could put my foot on to the top of the mounting block, creating an additional "step" with my leg to put her foot on to give her enough height to swing her right leg over in order to mount. This created a dilemma for Amy. Despite knowing that she was underweight, she feared that she would be too heavy for me to support her, and began to admonish herself for her inability to do it by herself. I suggested that we could experiment with how much weight she would be prepared to allow me to support, by gradually testing the strength of my "step" before actually mounting the horse. She agreed and we spent several minutes testing my support of her, with Amy increasing the weight that she lent on my leg each time. We paid attention to how this felt for her to be able to test it out first and she reported that she was surprised that I could take her weight and that she felt safer and calmer with each attempt. We continued this until Amy felt ready to mount, at which point she noticed how Spirit had remained patiently in place by the mounting block the entire time and expressed her gratitude and surprise that she was there, and that this level of support was available to her. Amy became tearful as she recognized how often she continues to struggle on her own for fear of being too much of a heavy burden for anyone else, even when help is available and offered.

With a deep exhale, Amy stepped up onto my leg and swung herself onto Spirit. I encouraged her to describe the physical sensations of being on the horse bareback, and to notice how Spirit was responding to her being on her back, and where and how she thought Spirit might want to be stroked. Amy began to stretch forward to pet Spirit on her neck. Spirit responded with turning her head toward Amy. When Amy stroked her on the other side, she turned the other way. Amy turned around to scratch Spirit on her rump, clearly relaxing in her body as she immersed herself into the experience. I asked if she would like to try lying down on her back, explaining that I would be right next to both of them for safety. Hesitantly, Amy began to lean backward. Reaching for my hand, she steadied herself as she lowered her back onto Spirit. With her legs astride the horse, this posture creates a deep stretch in the hip flexors as well as across the clavicle area as the shoulders rest on the horse. It is a position of complete surrender and of trust. If the horse should move, the client would feel every shift of motion. So it is with utmost care that this experience is offered, and usually only with clients who have built a relationship with the horse beforehand. Checking in with Amy, I asked her to make a statement about her experience in the moment.

> Amy: This feels incredible. I'm nervous but I know Spirit's got my back [...] literally! (Amy giggles as she says this). I can feel her breathing, and she's so calm. And I feel like I'm melting into her! (She giggles again). I feel so open. I feel so much gratitude for her right now.

The second stage of the HERD model of EFP of **release and expand** was initiated through processing Amy's dilemma in the moment of being "too much." Testing out first her own, then mine, and then Spirit's capacity to tolerate her fullness of being, allowed her to feel the experiential liberation of trusting herself, me, and her horse enough, while staying connected in the relationships, and opened her up to the possibility of living more fully.

This stage of the HERD model of EFP supports the releasing of psychological constriction and the expansion of the client's horizons, and is experienced as clients reach beyond boundaries to dismantle old barriers. Through releasing these internalized constraints, clients can begin to develop a more robust and expanded experience of themselves, and become more aware of the physical sensations of tension and restriction in their bodies. This leads to the full surrender and letting go of the "shoulds" in order to be fully present in the moment with the other. It is in this shared space with another that clients experience an alignment and gathering together of previously fragmented parts of themselves, and begin to develop a felt sense of their own authentic presence. Following this experience, Amy was also able to access a wider perspective of her lived relationships in her life; recognizing and showing gratitude for her family for sticking with her throughout her treatment, relapse after relapse. In the same way as she experimented with testing out my support, Amy reclaimed some of her own agency in acknowledging that she was making an effort in her recovery. This allowed her to not only release some long held negative beliefs about herself, but also take up more space in the world, expanding and reoccupying her own embodied space.

REVISITING THE LESSONS LEARNED

It is imperative for practitioners to understand that the HERD model of EFP is not a linear or static process. Through the lived experiences of our clients, it would be tempting to track the progress of clients based on which stage of the model they are at. In truth, some clients may appear to move through the whole cycle within one session, while others remain in one stage for a number of months, or dance between the stages. This does not mean that one is making more progress than the other; instead, we pay attention to the depth of learning from each stage.

I had been working with Amy for a year when my husband's job necessitated our relocation out of state. Amy had been making steady progress, and the multidisciplinary team at the eating disorders clinic had been preparing to discharge her. Our final session was marked by a celebratory trail ride through the woods as we reviewed her progress. Amy spoke of her growing confidence in taking up more space in the world, and becoming more visible in her relationships with others. Her ability to take charge and lead her horse and steer through obstacles on the trail ride was a testament to her progress. The trail ride was something that she had always yearned for but had not felt confident enough to do. So, I felt great pride in witnessing her confidence and empowered spirit.

BACK AND FORTH

Living with anorexia nervosa is a lonely existence. Social engagements, which often involve communal eating, are fraught with anxiety and purposefully avoided. Amy had become isolated from her peers and family, further confirming her view of herself as unworthy of attention. In the world of social media, this existential isolation is increasingly overcome by seeking out pro-anorexia support groups to find "thinspiration" that results in peer pressure like no other. This is the process through which Amy rapidly attached to and created her anorexic identity, where the awareness for the need to belong and relate to like-minded others catapulted her back into her relapse, time, and again. From an existential-humanistic perspective, it was here that I most needed to rely on my own ability to stay present and be available for connection within the relationship with Amy. From within the HERD model of EFP, and through Buber's I-thou approach to relating, I viewed her illness as an illness of her relations with the world. For Amy, as an individual suffering from anorexia, her relationship with the world, and herself, was through her way of being with (out) food. Duker and Slade, experts in the treatment of anorexia nervosa, suggest that for Amy, her

> *ability to restrict food has become not just the difference between being good or being bad, being a success or a failure. It has become the difference between being and not being. It has become [her] solution to being at all.*

Working with clients with anorexia nervosa requires an understanding of the depths of their despair. This includes their propensity for relapse, despite any apparent progress during their time in therapy. For this reason, the HERD model of EFP is particularly suited to those who may need to be reminded of their previous successes in therapy. By virtue of being living, breathing, and sentient beings who witnessed the client's journey and shared the embodied experiences of their endeavors, the horses are able to facilitate a client's return from relapse. This reminder of the importance of the intentionally relational aspect of sharing space allows for clients to reengage with the process of recovery.

A year after my departure, I returned to the area to deliver a workshop at the equine facility. The director at the eating disorders clinic heard that I would be in town and asked if I would have a session with Amy, who was back in treatment with her.

I watched Amy get out of the car, shoulders slumped forward, head lowered and eyes downcast, and wondered what had happened to her to trigger another relapse into the destructive cycle of anorexia. Amy stood before me feeling defeated and angry with herself and the world, believing that no one cared enough to notice her struggles. She was angry with me for leaving her a year ago. Now her friends had all left for college and she didn't want to admit to them that she was feeling left behind, so had withdrawn from any contact with them. Even her primary therapist had left the clinic, leaving her to start anew with someone else whom she didn't feel a connection with. She felt utterly abandoned and alone. Everything had changed and everyone else had moved on; even this herd of horses that she had felt so connected to previously had now doubled in size with new members since we had last worked together, and thus felt unfamiliar to her.

As we stood in the paddock, Amy began to describe her sense of futility, collapsing in on herself as she spoke. What began as a litany of reasons why she was unworthy of attention soon turned into her acknowledging the despair she was feeling in her isolation. She was convinced that once "out of sight, out of mind."

As she began to describe her fears, one by one, all six of the original herd members that she had worked with previously began to make their way over to us from the other side of the paddock where they had been grazing. One by one, they stood before her, sniffed, bowed their heads, and then stepped to one side to make room for the next. One by one, they greeted her and presented themselves to be available to work with her, connect with her, and be a shoulder to lean on for her. They stood in a circle facing her, waiting patiently. I asked her if she had noticed that all her old friends had come to greet her. She was uncertain and told me that the horses had come to see me and their presence had nothing to do with her. Quietly, I stepped away from them all until I was about 30 feet away, trusting that the horses would stay with her. As Amy reached out to each horse and greeted them in turn, her eyes shone with tears as she breathed in and remembered the authentic relationships she had made, where she could begin to believe that she mattered, that she had an impact on those around her, and that she was not alone.

Ultimately, Amy's story is a classic rendition of the importance of relationships and echoes the existential-humanistic and Gestalt principles that it is the relationship that heals. It offers the HERD practitioner a glimpse of the depth of work possible within the first two stages of the model, and highlights the power of the phenomenological and I-Thou approach.

For me, one of the most challenging aspects of being a therapist is in not knowing how the story plays out for many of my clients. There are some who will forever stand out in my memory, and each time my thoughts land on them, I take a moment to send out my heartfelt gratitude to them, and continued hope that they have found a way to thrive in the world. Amy's journey is one that I hold dearly in my heart, as her story captures the essence of my philosophical foundations; that by opening oneself to meeting another with grace, and holding space for the possibility of deep connection to occur, the most painful wounds can begin to heal, and light can enter through the cracks of the walls we have built to protect ourselves.

It is also a humbling experience to facilitate and witness this type of transformative process between clients. This next vignette offers a glimpse into the healing potential of EFP within the context of working with couples.

CASE STUDY 2: EMBODIED TOUCH

Mike and Angela were referred to me for EFP by Angela's primary therapist. After 5 years of individual therapy, Angela wanted to embark on some couples counseling. Married, with two children, aged 8 and 10, they had been struggling to connect physically and emotionally after Angela had confided with Mike 3 years previously about her childhood sexual trauma. Believing that telling Mike about the abuse that she had suffered would bring them closer, Angela felt hurt and betrayed that it had resulted in him distancing himself emotionally. Physically, the couple had not been sexually intimate for almost 2 years. Angela had suffered from depression for most of her adult life, and Mike felt responsible and helpless that he could not "make her happy." He also felt angry and frustrated that their once passionate relationship had dwindled to a perfunctory "kiss on the cheek" routine.

Angela was a petite woman, with delicate features and big blue eyes. She occupied very little space and carried herself with precision movements. Each gesture, motion, and expression was deliberate, concise, and quick. She clasped her hands together in front of her chest and sat with her shoulders hunched over. Her chin tilted down as she raised her eyes up at me with her eyes wide open, reminding me of a small bird watching out for danger. Mike, on the other hand, was solidly built. As a fitness enthusiast, he was a muscly, lean, 6 feet tall presence that towered over her petite frame. He had turned to going to the gym as an outlet for his sexual frustrations, and was meticulous about his workout routine and nutritional regime. His gestures were expansive and elaborate, waving his hand around to emphasize his point. He moved fluidly without restriction and took up the space around him with confidence.

Despite the difficulties they were experiencing, Mike and Angela were deeply committed to each other and believed that they would be able to find a way back toward a more connected relationship. They had come to the EFP sessions with an open mind and were eager to learn more about how they could become "unstuck" in their relationship.

After completing our initial check-in and safety protocol, I invited them to enter into the herd to get to know the horses. Reminding them to pay attention to their own breath and internal dialogue of what they were observing in the horses, we stepped into the paddock where the horses were grazing.

Mike immediately began to walk up toward one of the mares, approaching her head on as she grazed. As he got closer, he reached out his hand to stroke her between the ears. The mare, Tess, lifted her head abruptly and took several steps away from him. In response, Mike stepped forward and again reached out to pet her. Once again, Tess backed away. Again, Mike approached her, this time saying, "Aw, I just want to say hello and give you some love," before patting her on her neck. At this, Tess spun around and trotted away. Meanwhile, Angela stood to one side observing their interaction, seemingly frozen to the spot.

Mike:	Well that didn't work. She obviously didn't like me.
Angela:	She didn't have much time to get to know you.
Mike:	She did! I gave her lots of attention.
Angela:	Maybe it wasn't the right kind of attention.

At this, Angela let out a big sigh and tears filled her eyes. I asked her to describe what she had witnessed between Mike and Tess.

Angela:	He kept coming at her even though she wasn't interested. And he did it so abruptly it probably startled her.
Me:	How do you think she would've preferred to be approached?
Angela:	More slowly and less demanding. More on her own terms.

I invited Angela to go and connect with Tess in her own way. Looking around, she spotted a tree near to where Tess was now grazing. Slowly, she walked up to the tree and leant with her back against it facing the pasture. Tess was now about 10 feet away, facing her with her head down, still grazing. Mike and I stood a little further away observing. After about a minute, Mike called out to Angela, "I don't think she knows you want her attention." Angela shrugged, but continued focusing her attention on Tess. Another minute passed. Mike was getting impatient, "What are you waiting for? Get her attention," he said. "I'm waiting for her to be ready," said Angela as she began to cry. As she said this, Tess lifted up her head, looked directly at Angela, and began to walk towards her.

Being a Percheron cross, Tess was a big-framed horse. At 15.2hh, she wasn't particularly tall, but she had a solid, broad chest, wide back, and big head. Her deep soulful eyes and steady gaze provided her with an undeniable presence. She stood in front of Angela and lowered her head so that she was eye-level to her. Angela slowly reached out and began stroking Tess on her neck.

Me:	What would you like to say to Tess?
Angela:	Thank you for letting me know you were ready.
Me:	What would you like to say to Mike?
Angela:	I need you to be patient with me when you want my attention. When you want to be physically intimate. You can't rush me because that startles me.
Mike:	I don't mean to startle you. Is that what you think I do with you? I just want you to know that I want you!
Angela:	Sometimes, and I know it's frustrating for you when I reject your advances too. When I know that you are expecting something from me, it makes me tense and nervous.
Mike:	And when you tense up, I already feel rejected.

This interaction opened up into an exploration of how Mike and Angela felt on an embodied level in their frustrations and fear of intimacy. I encouraged Mike to follow Angela's lead on how to connect with Tess in a way that felt less demanding on her, and worked on attending to a felt sense of openness to connection without expectations. We focused on breathing, noticing where they held tension in their bodies, and paid attention to the sounds and sensations of standing in the open pasture with Tess by their side.

Mike stood by the tree next to Angela with his eyes closed and breathed deeply. Telling Tess that he was available to connect with her and that he was willing to wait until she was ready, Mike relaxed against the tree. After a few minutes, Tess made her way over to him and began nudging him in the chest with her muzzle, sniffing and moving her lips against the fabric of his jacket. Mike smiled and looked at Angela and asked her to show him what to do next. At this invitation, Angela took his hand and guided him in stroking Tess gently on her chest. Tess, in turn, stretched out her neck and lifted her head, exposing more of her chest. With each movement we paid attention to what meaning Mike and Angela made of Tess' response.

This moment-by-moment discovery of what they concluded was Tess' way of expressing how and where she liked to be touched continued for the rest of the session. They took turns in scratching her, stroking her, and massaging her. They experimented with different pressure and techniques and watched her responses to see which she seemed to like more. They played with stroking her simultaneously from either side, and stayed curious to her responses. Supporting them to engage with Tess on her terms, allowed Mike to recognize how he triggered Angela's trauma response through his insistence in getting her attention, and enabled Angela to be clearer about her boundaries and desires. Seeing Tess' enjoyment of being stroked and petted, Angela commented that perhaps this was something they could do with each other too, and experiment with what was tolerable for her in terms of touch.

Mike commented that Angela's way of touching Tess seemed very timid in comparison to his own. I shared my observations in terms of how I saw each of them occupying the space around them. Angela immediately connected this to her sense of needing to stay small and not draw attention to herself as a result of her childhood trauma. In turn, Mike explained that in his family of origin as one of six siblings, he had to make himself visible in order to get attention, and his expansiveness was his way of meeting that need. This awareness brought about a shift in the way that the couple was able to make meaning from each other's relational embodied interactions. Mike admitted that due to Angela's more subtle ways of communicating bodily, that he found it hard to know when she might want physical intimacy, or indeed what she might need. Angela acknowledged that over the years, she had let Mike take responsibility for initiating any physical contact and realized that she was unsure of what she needed. She commented that by seeing Tess' response to their touch made her realize that she didn't give Mike much feedback as to what she needed or liked. Seeing Tess respond with such obvious and immediate feedback supported her wish to express more clearly her own desires.

It was also important for Angela that Tess was engaging with them voluntarily and was not tied or confined while they interacted with her. This freedom of choice resonated strongly with Angela and supported her to express her need to hold her boundaries, and recognize that unlike during her childhood, she now had choice and ownership of her embodied self. Mike acknowledged that he had distanced himself for fear of her feeling that he would intentionally force her to do something she did not want to, but that he missed the connection that they previously shared.

This dialogue enabled the couple to deepen their connection with each other in a truly I-Thou way of relating. By staying curious to Tess' responses to them, and subsequently to each other, they ventured into a space of mutuality.

This vignette illustrates clearly the **Deepening** stage of the HERD model of EFP. Exploring Mike and Angela's differences in their embodied ways of being-in-the-world supported them to listen intently to their own process. The development of their feelings of intentionality and personal agency through their interactions with Tess brought about the confirmation of their inner experiences. This enabled them to own their truth and solidify an internal sense of themselves. With this clarity, they were able to approach each other with a fuller sense of integrity, empathy, and openness with regards to the struggles they were experiencing in their marriage. Through this process, they were able to sink deeper into the support available from each other and begin to heal the ruptures.

I worked with Mike and Angela for almost a year in weekly sessions. The theme that they held onto throughout our time together was one of "space": how much space was given or taken in the relationship, both physically and emotionally; how little space Angela occupied when feeling unsafe; how much space Mike occupied when he felt frustrated; and the continuous monitoring and self-regulation required to negotiate the space between them. We worked with Tess in many sessions, but also with the other members of the herd, both individually and collectively, and took care to observe the differences between them. Mike and Angela were able to make meaning from their observations of the relationships within the herd. In particular, they were fascinated by the intentionality and boundaries they witnessed within the herd, and took great care to pay attention to that within their own relationship in each moment.

This case study also highlights the importance of the HERD practitioner's understanding of working with clients with trauma and attachment issues. Both Mike and Angela described disruptions in their attachment process. Added to this, Angela's history of childhood sexual trauma, where it was necessary to be careful to not retraumatize her in the embodied work we did, required me to track even more closely than usual her embodied responses during our sessions. An embodied approach to trauma often takes clients to a deeper release of trauma more quickly than other approaches. Going deeper and faster is not the aim. Going deeper with awareness within a safe container is preferable to simply unearthing the trauma with nowhere for it to go. This can often leave clients feeling unsupported and retraumatized.

The HERD approach emphasizes the existential-humanistic embodiment of being "a part of, or apart from" those around us. In their journey with the herd, Mike and Angela were able to experience and embody the constantly shifting parameters of where one feels a sense of belonging; both with the horses and with each other. Their journey captures the essence of the deepening stage of the HERD model of EFP, where they were able to sink into a mutually supportive embrace, and was a testament to the love and commitment they held for each other.

CASE STUDY 3: THE LANGUAGE OF LOVE

The Jacobs family was referred to me through an outpatient treatment center specializing in adolescents with at-risk behaviors. The treatment center focuses on the preservation of the family through at-home intensive family therapy. Therapists work with the families to prevent out-of-home placements at residential centers, or to reunify family members following residential treatment. By the time the families are referred to me, the "identified clients" (the adolescents) are either at the beginning of their journey home from treatment or at the last resort before being sent away. Presenting issues include severe depression, active suicidal ideation, drug/alcohol/gaming/gambling addictions, anxiety, and intergenerational trauma.

The Jacobs were a family of four: mom (Alison), dad (Billy), and two daughters, Melody and Suzy. Billy was a pastor and Alison was a stay-at-home mom. The family had enlisted the center's services for Melody. At 15 years old, Melody had already been in residential treatment three times for attempted suicide. The first incident occurred when she was 12, and involved her sending suicide notes via texts to five of her classmates one morning, saying that she was going to end her life that day so would not be in school. The second attempt occurred on her 13th birthday after an argument with her mom when she was told she could not attend a rock concert. This time, she went through all the medicine cabinets and collected up all the medication she could find and locked herself in the bathroom. Her final, and most recent, attempt occurred 4 weeks before our session, and involved her cutting her wrist with a pair of scissors. The cut was relatively superficial and did not require stitches, but her parents were alarmed by what they deemed to be her most serious attempt to date. After each episode, Melody had been hospitalized and referred to a psychiatrist. Each time, when asked for her reasons for wanting to commit suicide, she responded by saying that she did not want to be part of this family anymore and that she would rather die than have to live with them. This was a phrase that she repeated often to her parents and in front her of younger sister.

Suzy was 4 years younger than Melody, and had compensated for what she called her sister's "troubles" by adopting the "good girl" persona in the family. She excelled in her studies, was compliant with her parents, and never gave her parents cause for concern. Her relationship with Melody was one of tolerance and protectiveness. Suzy was highly attuned to Melody's mood changes and would attempt to soothe her when she became agitated or upset. She seemed to accept that Melody needed more of her parent's attention, and did not appear to begrudge that. Suzy was, however, extremely hurt by Melody's declarations of not wanting to be part of the family, and was frightened by the latest suicide attempts.

When the family arrived at the barn for their first session, Melody was first to the gate and introduced herself to me exuberantly. Suzy stood behind her avoiding eye contact with me. Mom and dad walked up slowly as I held the gate open for them. We stood outside the barn and went through our preliminary introductions and the HERD Safety Protocol. Melody immediately informed me that she was experienced around horses and knows how to ride. Her mom, Alison, corrected her by telling me that she was exaggerating, as was her tendency, and in fact had only been trail riding a couple of times in her life. Suzy, on the other hand, voiced that she was nervous around horses so really didn't want to participate. Billy responded to her by threatening to ground her for a week if she did not take part. Suzy acquiesced and stepped into the barn.

What struck me the most about the family as they made their way inside was the difference in their energetic presence. Melody was excitable, bouncy in her step, and chatty. Her voice was loud and her gestures were rapid and expansive, and she appeared to keep an extensive bubble of personal space around her, never moving in close proximity to the rest of the family. Suzy and her parents, on the other hand, moved as one. They clumped together with very little space between them and collectively took up less space than Melody by herself. They moved slowly and tentatively, with small and abrupt gestures. They spoke softly and quietly, taking time to consider their words carefully before uttering them aloud. Melody seemed to speak without a filter, and provided a continuous vocal stream of consciousness.

When asked what each of them were hoping for from the session, Melody took the lead to express her desire for experiencing something as a family that was different to their usual talking therapy sessions. She was adamant that she wanted to find a way to move forward in their lives without her destructive behaviors blocking their path toward true connection. As she spoke, her eyes darted around the barn, and she shifted her weight from one foot to the other, swinging her arms around from side to side. I became aware of my own embodied response to her as one of needing to keep my distance. As I listened to her speak, I felt like she had memorized a brochure for family therapy. Something felt amiss as her words were incongruent with her bodily expressions. The rest of the family agreed that they were hoping for an experience that would unify them. Alison commented that they were eager to "help prevent Melody from destroying herself." Billy wanted Melody to tell them how to they could help her. Suzy hoped that they could collectively "make Melody feel better."

When working with families, I find that they often arrive with a focus on the identified client as the one that needs to be "fixed." Not only does this create even more distance between the already struggling adolescent and the rest of the family, but it also positions them as the root cause of all the issues that the family is facing. Working from an existential-humanistic and Gestalt perspective, I regard the family situation in the totality of their experiences, where each member contributes to, and makes an impact on, the family dynamics as a whole. Every action or inaction creates a ripple effect through the family. That is to say, that it is not possible to not make an impact.

So when I witness this process of placing the emphasis on "fixing" the identified client, with the unacknowledged and nonverbal collusion that one person is to blame for the family's struggles, I will gently point out that healing and connection does not depend solely on that one family member to change their way of being-in-the-family. Instead, it requires commitment and willingness by everyone involved to shift their perspectives to focus on how they all interact with each other.

This exchange took place just after we had entered the herd. The two geldings, Isaac and Freeman, had slowly been making their way from across the paddock towards us together. As they got closer, they split off from each other. Isaac stood facing Melody about 6 feet away, and Freeman meandered across to the rest of the family and began to insert himself into the space between Alison and Billy, who stepped aside to make room for him. Once Freeman made his way safely between the two parents, he turned and walked toward Suzy. By now, Allison had moved and was standing in close proximity to Suzy. Freeman walked forward and inserted himself in between mom and daughter, forcing them to step further apart from each other. The family was now evenly spread out in a semi-circle in the paddock and the horses went back to grazing.

I asked them what meaning they made of the horses' maneuvers. Melody was the first to respond, and commented that she thought Isaac didn't want to get too close to anyone, as he had remained at arm's length the whole time. She thought that Freeman was more sociable, and maybe a "troublemaker" in the way that he had pushed everyone else around. Alison agreed, and noticed that Freeman had made sure to spread everyone out equally. At this, Suzy chimed in with "Maybe he thinks we should include Melody more, because she was standing all by herself to start with."

This interaction flowed into an exploration of the existing family dynamics where Melody keeps to herself, not wanting to be part of the family, and how this impacts on everyone else. I reminded them that their hope at the beginning was to have a unifying experience as a family, and invited them to pay attention to how they were feeling as we proceeded. I suggested that they might want to find a way to meet and greet the horses together, as a family unit, and observe the horses' responses to them doing that. Offering them the freedom to decide between them how they might want to do that, I stepped aside and observed their next steps as they negotiated who they wanted to go up to first.

Alison and Suzy wanted to meet Freeman. Melody wanted to go to Isaac. Billy said he didn't have a preference and would go with the majority vote.

I watched as Melody's demeanor changed. Her initial brightness diminished, and her shoulders slumped forward. Sticking her hands in her jacket pockets, she shuffled across the paddock behind the rest of the family as they headed toward Freeman. As they stood around him, Freeman lifted his head from grazing and sniffed each of them in turn. Alison, Billy, and Suzy stepped in closer toward Freeman and began to pet him on his neck and shoulders. Melody stood on the periphery as they did this and looked over at Isaac. The others were absorbed in their interaction with Freeman, marveling at his musculature, his size, and facial expressions as they stroked him, seemingly unaware that Melody was not part of the experience. Meanwhile, Melody began to drift away from them, slowly but surely, meandering over to Isaac who lifted up his head to greet her by gently breathing out in her face. She smiled and began to stroke him. I looked back across to the rest of the family who were still focused on Freeman.

> Me: I'd just like you to pay attention on what's happening right now. I notice that Melody has moved away from everyone. What happened to doing this all together?
>
> Billy: Well, we're all together, but I guess she chose to walk away from us, as usual.

At this, Melody tensed up her body and held her breath. Spinning round to glare at the rest of the family, she declared that they didn't want her to be there anyway, so there was no point in her being there with them.

> Suzy: You're the one that walked away. We didn't tell you to.
> Alison: Yes, we were all here doing this together and you didn't want to.
> Melody: Why would I? This is what always happens if I don't agree with you. You all just start ganging up against me!
> Alison: That's not true. You always want to go off by yourself to do your own thing.
> Melody: I hate this family. I don't want to be here, and I don't want to be part of this family. I'd rather die!

Melody began walking away from the horses toward the paddock gate. I asked her to wait, and to give us a chance to process what had just happened. She stopped and spun around, folded her arms across her chest and glared at her family. I turned and addressed the rest of the family, and asked if anyone had noticed that Melody had drifted off by herself while they were petting Freeman. They looked at each other, surprised, and then looked down at their feet as they shook their heads.

> Alison: I guess we were so absorbed with Freeman; I didn't pay attention to what Melody was doing. I thought she was right here with us. I'm sorry, Melody.

This awareness brought about a profound shift in Alison and Billy's perspective. We began to explore how they communicate within the family to let Melody know that they want to be with her, and that they want her to be part of the family without shifting the responsibility onto her. When invited to find a different way of relating to each other, the family was able to see that they do gang up against Melody, albeit unintentionally. They were able to refer back to their experience of Freeman's maneuvers and interpreted it as his way of making sure that each member of the family took responsibility for the cohesiveness of the family, and to not leave Melody out. We worked on finding a different way of communicating the underlying message that they wanted the other person to hear in the moment, in an effort to not become critical. For example, instead of saying "You're going off to do your own thing," to say, "We want you to be part of this family." For Melody, instead of saying "I don't want to be part of this family," to say, "I'm feeling left out." Melody was able to express to the rest of the family that she needed to hear that they loved her, and that they wanted to be around her, and not just to be seen as the "troublemaker." As Alison and Billy began to protest that they have told her that, Suzy intervened, and pointed out that there was a difference between saying a perfunctory "Love you, good night" to saying it with meaning. She reminded the family of Billy's sermon from the previous Sunday when he said "Love is a language rooted in action," and that they did not demonstrate an action-based love language in the family.

As the family worked through these statements and found ways to express what they were feeling to each other, Freeman and Isaac began to move closer. Skirting around the perimeter, the horses walked around the family in ever decreasing concentric circles. As the horses moved, the family members adjusted themselves to make room for the horses. I asked if they were aware of what the horses were doing. "They're encouraging us to stand closer together as a family!" exclaimed Suzy. Melody was delighted by this insight and spontaneously reached across to Suzy and hugged her. The session ended with the family committing to paying more attention to more intentional expressions of love through action. Additionally, they were able to take responsibility for their part in the family's struggles in a way that did not place blame on Melody.

A few weeks after this session, I had a follow-up meeting with the family's primary therapist from the clinic. She reported that the family was thriving in their new commitment to each other in finding alternative ways of expressing themselves through nonblaming language. Melody had commented to her that the EFP session had allowed her to feel more at-home in herself and with her family because they had discovered a "love-based language" with each other.

This vignette clearly demonstrates the fourth stage of the HERD model of EFP of Coming Home to Relationships. Through noticing the horses' interactions with the family, and an exploration of the meaning the clients made of that process, a different way of being-in-the family was possible. Facilitating the shift in perspectives for both the individual members in the family, and the family's totality of their experience allowed them to find a deeper connection with each other that was based in the here-and-now. This present moment awareness supported the family to find their authentic voices, individually and collectively, so that they could communicate from a place of inner yearning and meet each other in a way that honored their own experiences. This moved them away from their habitual ways of being within the family and empowered them to take ownership of their intentions and desires. Through their love-based language, the family found a common communicative home and the beginnings of a return to self and relationships.

CASE STUDY 4: ONE BREATH, ONE MOVEMENT

When I first met Chris, he was 9 years old. He had been referred to me through a child and adolescent therapist with whom he had been working with for about a year. His primary therapist felt that EFP sessions would help him to open up more about his felt experiences, as he had been struggling to articulate himself in their sessions. We initially arranged a series of weekly sessions for a 12-week period, the aim of which was to ascertain whether Chris required more intensive treatment at a residential program.

Chris was diagnosed with ADHD at the age of 4, and had recently received additional diagnoses of severe anxiety and Tourette's Syndrome 3 months prior to our meeting. He was a middle child with two brothers who were 3 years apart on either side. Before I began working with him, I met with both Chris and his mother, who reported that she had always had a hard time bonding with him. His mother, Shelly, had suffered from post-natal depression with all three boys, but had a particularly severe episode with Chris. Shelly struggled with what she experienced as Chris' incessant need for attention and high-energy levels, stating that she began suspecting that he had ADHD when he turned 3 years old. She described how he would constantly run up to her and launch himself into her for hugs and physical attention, and how he could not sit still for any length of time. When his younger brother was born, Chris exhibited extreme separation anxiety and would not leave her side. This anxiety had recently spiked to include school refusal and the development of a facial and phonic tic that resulted in his Tourette's diagnosis. Shelly reported that the tic caused him additional anxiety and had become a vicious cycle that they could not free him from. There did not seem to be any correlation between the tic and particular activities.

This assessment session took place at the barn where I met with clients. It was a beautiful day, so we had taken a seat on the bleachers next to the outdoor arena. While Shelly and I talked, Chris sat at the other end of the bleachers from us. There was a show jumping practice session under way in the arena and Chris was mesmerized. For the entire duration of the intake, he sat glued to the action in the arena, never once taking his eyes off the proceedings. His eyes were bright and he leaned forward eagerly as riders approached each jump. Having kept my eye on Chris during our conversation, I commented that I had yet to witness his tic. Shelly seemed surprised as it had apparently been particularly prominent that day.

Armed with the information that Shelly had provided, I wanted to spend some time with Chris one-on-one. I asked Shelly to stay on the bleachers while I took Chris to meet the herd. Contrary to Shelly's description of his separation anxiety, Chris eagerly followed me toward the barn away from his mother. As we walked away, I could hear Shelly asking him if he felt okay to go with me on his own, or whether he wanted her to go with him. I was certain that he had heard her, but Chris made no response and continued walking alongside me, with his eyes forward and a bounce in his step. He started telling me how much he loves animals, in particular dogs and cats, and that he had never been around horses before, but that he was sure that they would be amazing friends to have. As we approached the barn, I explained the HERD Safety Protocol to him. Chris paid close attention to my explanation and was able to repeat back to me the safety agreement without hesitation.

We entered the herd and spent a few minutes taking in the scene. In an effort to ease him into his surroundings, I asked Chris what he saw. He responded with a meticulous description of the horses, trees, and paddock, and even included sounds that he was aware of. I felt his energetic presence to be completely rooted in the moment, engaged and intentional in his desire to be with the horses. As we walked a little closer to the grazing herd, he stopped, closed his eyes, and inhaled deeply.

Chris: It smells so good here. I could just stay here forever!
Me: Take your time and stay right there for a while.
Chris: But aren't I supposed to be doing something?
Me: Seems to me like you are doing exactly what you need.
Chris: I think I am!

Closing his eyes once more, Chris continued to stand in the middle of the paddock breathing deeply. His shoulders relaxed, and his jaw unlocked. As he tilted his head up to the sky and smiled, I stood and witnessed this young boy immerse himself in the beauty of the moment, marveling at his ability to stay embodied and present, and felt baffled by the distinct mismatch of his mother's description of him. I put that thought to one side to ponder over later, and took in a deep breath to recenter myself to be with Chris.

I invited Chris to play the "I notice" game with his eyes closed. He began with noticing the smell of the trees and grass, the wind on his face, the sounds of the horses grazing, and the birds in the trees. As he spoke, two of the mares in the herd began to make their way over toward us. I asked Chris to open his eyes to take in their arrival, and he smiled as he watched the mares approach him.

Buttercup, a palomino pony, walked up to Chris and nudged him on his shoulder with her muzzle. Chris frowned and stepped to one side. Buttercup advanced again and repeated her nudging. Chris, again, stepped away.

Buttercup advanced once more and nudged him. Again, Chris stepped away without a word. In that moment, I noticed his facial tic.

Me:	How do you feel right now?
Chris:	Like she's pushing me around. I just wanted to make friends but she keeps shoving me.
Me:	What do you think she's saying?
Chris:	That I need to get out of her way.
Me:	How are you in her way?
Chris:	I don't know. I'm always in the way.

He held his breath as his eyes filled with tears. Turning away from me, he wiped his tears away with his sleeve and looked down at the ground. His shoulders tensed as I felt him try to contain himself. Before I could respond, Coco the miniature mare, trotted over and stood in between Chris and Buttercup. As Buttercup attempted to skirt around Coco, the mini-mare blocked her advances toward Chris. Buttercup advanced once more, and Coco pinned her ears at her and stopped her in her tracks. I asked Chris what he made of the mares' interactions.

Chris:	The little one is keeping the big one away.
Me:	She is. How do you feel about that?
Chris:	I like it. She's protecting me from the bully.

During this interaction, Chris' facial tic appeared several times. His eyes twitched and he blinked rapidly. He tilted his head abruptly from side to side. He vocalized a quiet "Oh, oh" as he tilted his head. His breathing became shallow and his fists clenched together. I encouraged him to take a deep breath before proceeding, needing him to find his ground as I knew that this would be a revealing moment for him in our process. Gently, I asked him who Buttercup reminded him of. He shook his head and pursed his lips. I waited. After a few moments he took a breath. Keeping his eyes downcast he answered quietly, "My mom."

My heart went out to this sweet, gentle child. I felt a surge of protective-ness for him and a wave of sadness as I pieced together the contrast between my experience of him and his mother's description. I realized that the work in this instance was to repair the rupture between mother and child. Shelly's post-natal depression and the interruption in Chris' attachment process were evident in the way they experienced each other. Chris' experience of himself as always being in the way was an embodied one that reflected his mother's ambivalence toward him during her post-natal depression. This ambivalence had clearly continued past her depression and had become an habitual atti-tude she held toward him. It was an accurate assessment on his part of her embodied way of relating to him.

Continuing with the session, I asked Chris what he'd like to say to Buttercup.

Chris:	Please don't get mad at me. I don't know what you want.

As he said this, Coco moved out of the way and Buttercup walked over and stopped about 15 feet in front of Chris. She stood there quietly without nudging him.

Me:	Do you think she's mad at you right now?
Chris:	No. I don't think so anymore. But now I don't know what she wants.
Me:	What do *you* want?
Chris:	I want to give her a hug.
Me:	Would you like to try and see how she responds?
Chris:	Okay. I'd like that. But only if you don't think she'll get mad.
Me:	I can't promise, but I think it's worth a try?

Chris nodded. As we began to walk toward Buttercup, Chris reached over and held my hand. I gave his hand a little squeeze of encouragement and guided him toward the horse. I positioned myself slightly behind Chris, still holding his hand as he reached Buttercup's side. Chris reached out and petted her. As he stroked her, he let go of my hand and let out a big sigh. I encouraged him to reach up with both arms to give the horse a hug. Buttercup lowered her head and draped it over the boy's back. Chris leaned into the mare and buried his face in her shoulder. Coming up for air, he smiled broadly. We wrapped up the session with him giving Buttercup one more hug, during which she blew out on the top of his head making him giggle. Throughout this interaction, his facial tic had not surfaced. He walked away with a bounce in his step, eager to relay what had happened to his mom.

As we approached his mom, he sprinted toward her and threw his arms around her. With a sinking heart, I watched as she pushed him to one side, telling him to calm down and not jump on her. Chris' entire body slumped and his tic returned. With Chris present, I addressed his mother and told her that he had done really well, and that he'd been a really good boy with me; that he'd listened well and had paid attention, and that I was looking forward to getting to know him more. He smiled shyly at me. Shelly expressed her surprise. I told her I was genuinely impressed by his ability to articulate what he'd been feeling, and his willingness to engage with me in his process. As Chris got into the car, I asked if I could speak with Shelly out of earshot.

I enquired as to whether she would be open to having mother-son sessions with Chris, and explained that I felt that the work that needed to be done was to repair the disconnect between them. As I spoke, Shelly became tearful. She agreed that she had always felt disconnected to Chris, but didn't know how to be with him without feeling irritated by him. She desperately wanted to connect with him, but felt stuck in a downward spiral. She felt relieved to know that there might be a way out, and we agreed to move forward with joint sessions.

Over the next few months, I worked with Shelly and Chris in attuning to each other. For both of them, I paid attention to their habitual reactions to each other. In one session, I had asked Chris to walk across the paddock to fetch a halter for one of the horses. As Shelly watched him walking away, I noticed her exhaling. Asking her to pay attention to her breathing, she acknowledged that every time Chris left her side, she felt a sense of relief. Whenever she felt he needed her, she was reminded of the panic that she felt during her post-natal depression, where she felt she couldn't give him what he needed, and instead felt irritated by his neediness. This was then followed by feelings of guilt and shame, and it was this downward spiral that kept her stuck in her relationship with Chris. At the same time, she also desperately wanted to connect with him, but opening herself up to his neediness felt too overwhelming.

She finished telling me this as Chris returned with the halter. They had picked Buttercup, the palomino mare that had initially reminded Chris of his mom, to work with in this session. I invited them to go into the paddock together to go and put Buttercup's halter on her and lead her into the round pen. They accomplished this task easily, with Shelly allowing Chris to lead the way while she trailed slowly behind him. Having led Buttercup into the round pen, I suggested that they take her halter off and allow her the freedom to roam as she pleased. Upon being released, Buttercup circled the round pen, breathing in her surroundings before coming to a halt next to Chris.

Chris smiled at Buttercup and reached out to pet her on her neck. We had spent a few sessions grooming and petting the horses, breathing with them, and attending to shifts in their energy in relation to Chris and Shelly. They were now familiar with breathing deeply as a way of attending to their own emotional regulation. Now, Chris turned to his mom and asked her if she wanted to pet Buttercup with him. She nodded and stepped up to Buttercup next to Chris and they began to stroke her on her neck and belly. I noticed that Shelly's movements were faster and more abrupt than Chris', who was taking his time to stroke the horse in long fluid motions. I intervened and asked them to stand on opposite sides of Buttercup and invited them to synchronize their strokes with each other. I asked them to pay attention to Buttercup's responses to see if they could tell what she liked or didn't like.

Shelly had commented previously that she could feel herself physically relaxing as she petted the horses. She was happy to experiment with the synchronized petting, and Chris was eager to do something with his mom. His face lit up as they began to stroke the horse, but soon his facial and phonic tic began to surface. I asked him how he was feeling, and he responded that he didn't like not being able to see what his mom was doing, and that he was worried that he was doing it wrong. While Shelly was tall enough to look over Buttercup's back to see Chris to match his movements, he was not tall enough to see her. We spent some time figuring out the best way to communicate between them on how they were going to stroke the horse. At Shelly's suggestion, they began stroking at the top of Buttercup's neck in one fluid motion down to her hip. After several attempts, they were still struggling to synchronize their movements. Buttercup, in the meantime, had been standing still to receive their petting, but as Chris became more agitated, she turned her head toward him and nudged his arm.

> Chris: I think she's telling me to move over.
> Shelly: I think she's right. You might need to move down a little so that you can reach her hip when you stroke her from top to tail.
> Chris: Maybe we can count as we stroke so that we get there at the same time?

Buttercup nudged Chris again. He giggled and said he thought that she agreed. So they began to stroke her once more. They agreed to a count of five to get from her neck to her hip. After a couple of attempts, they began to relax into the motion and were in synch with each other. I suggested that they add another element to the game by paying attention to their breath as they stroked, and to aim for one breath, one movement. Breathing in before they began stroking, and exhaling as they stroked. I noticed Shelly watch Chris closely in order to stay synchronized. Her face softened and she smiled. Chris looked up at his mother and saw her watching him and smiled in return. His facial and phonic tic subsided. I gave them a few minutes to repeat this experience before asking them what they were feeling.

> Chris: I like it that mom is paying attention to me as well as Buttercup.
> Shelly: I like seeing you so calm and relaxed. I like feeling this calm and relaxed too!
> Chris: I like you calm and relaxed!

Shelly looked at me and asked if she could stop petting Buttercup. Chris' shoulders slumped and he looked down at the ground.

> Shelly: Don't look sad. I want to stop so I can come over to your side to give you a hug.

I will never forget the look on that young boy's face. He looked up at his mom with such surprise and delight. As Shelly walked in front of Buttercup, he turned and waited patiently for his mom to reach him. Shelly scooped Chris up and enveloped him in a tight hug and began to cry. Turning to me she whispered, "I need to do this more. I'm ready to give him what he needs." As they hugged each other, Buttercup walked in a circle around them before standing behind Chris and placing her head behind his back. "She's got your back kid," said Shelly. "I've got your back too," she added.

As we processed this interaction, I supported them to describe what they had experienced. This was subsequently referred to in later sessions as "The moment with Buttercup." Shelly was able to articulate how important it was for her to feel in synch with Chris. It allowed her to not feel overwhelmed by what she imagined he might need from her, and supported her to be able to see the simplicity of his requests. For her, Buttercup's response to her hugging Chris was taken as an act of approval. Chris in turn, was able to make meaning of his experiences with Buttercup through a growing awareness that his mom was beginning to understand more of what he wanted, and was available to provide him comfort when he needed, so that he no longer felt that he was always in the way.

A few years after I worked with Shelly and Chris, I received a letter from Shelly. In it, she thanked me for the work we did together. She wanted me to know that Chris was now about to start high school and was thriving. He was maturing into a confident and sociable young man, and she was very proud of him. While life had presented them with some challenges, they had been able to work through times when they became disconnected by referring to the moment with Buttercup of "One breath, one movement" to ascertain their needs, and to figure out how to meet them. Shelly wrote, "the experience was so profound for me. To be able to slow down and tune in to myself and then find him, and have the horse acknowledge it was huge."

This vignette illustrates the final stage of the HERD model of EFP of **integration**. When we experience something new and profound, whether it is a deeper understanding of ourselves, or our loved ones, the emotions that reveal themselves in the moment may fade away if there is no integration. This final stage is instrumental in supporting our clients to move out into the world while holding onto their experiences in therapy. It is here that they translate their experiences with us into something meaningful in their everyday lives. By encouraging clients to mindfully recall their experiences in an embodied way, we support them to fully absorb their experiences so that they become a lasting, embodied memory.

Working with Shelly and Chris, my focus was on repairing the ruptured attachment process caused by Shelly's post-natal depression. Through tracking their bodily process and continuously paying attention to their breathing, I watched for their outbreath after each "a-ha" moment as a sign of experiential integration. Encouraging them to describe in detail their experiences in the moment allowed for a phenomenological exploration of what and how meanings were made in their encounters with the horses. Chris' attachment to Buttercup, which began on rocky ground, was a parallel to his relationship with his mother. In supporting his connection with Buttercup, we were able to transfer his feelings toward her to Shelly. Likewise, in seeing Buttercup's responses to Chris, Shelly was able to let go of some of her fixed gestalt responses to him and find an alternative approach to their relationship.

This case study also clearly demonstrates the full progression of all five stages of the HERD model of EFP. From the beginning, we focused on Sharing Space. Chris' perception of himself as always being in the way in relation to Shelly was an accurate embodied experience. For Shelly to witness Chris' anxiety around her reactions to him allowed her to clearly see her part in the process, rather than placing the sole responsibility on Chris for changing his behavior. As we worked with the horses, over time, Chris and Shelly were both able to Release and Expand their long held restrictions and psychological constrictions. For Chris, his introjections led to extreme anxiety that was manifested in his facial and phonic tic. He began to tune into his bodily self as an embodied reoccupation and toward an embodied emotional regulation. For Shelly, she was able to let go of some of the guilt and shame that she had carried from her post-natal depression and widened her perspective of Chris and what their relationship might be like. This led to the Deepening of their relationship with each other as they brought themselves more fully and authentically into the relationship. This Deepening was facilitated with Buttercup as a conduit for communicating more clearly, and as an immediate feedback mechanism as they worked together. As they began to take more risks in the relationship, they were able to meet each other more fully in what they needed in an I-Thou manner. The presence (or absence) of Chris' facial and phonic tic also provided an embodied barometer for ascertaining his anxiety levels, and his ability to step into deeper contact with his mom. Through this, they were able to Come Home to the relationship and reoccupy their embodied self as well as take in more of the other and their environment. The final stage of integration supported them to take the experiential learning out into their everyday lives.

CASE STUDY 5: INTEGRATING THE HERD MODEL OF EFP WITH HUMANISTIC PLAY THERAPY

This case study offers a synthesis of the key concepts within the HERD model of EFP and Humanistic Play Therapy (HPT) and demonstrates that they are compatible modalities for working with children.

What Is Humanistic Play Therapy?

Humanistic Play Therapy (HPT) originated from the work of Virginia Axline in the 1940s and is a client-centered approach to therapy adapted for children and adolescents. HPT focuses on building a secure relationship between the therapist and client in order to empower them to express himself/herself authentically in each moment, thus honoring their phenomenal world. Viewing the supportive relationship as the key for growth and healing, the client utilizes play to make contact with the therapist in a way that is safe for the child. According to Bratton and Ray, leading HPT practitioners, underpinning HPT are key concepts of (a) the importance of the therapist-client relationship, (b) the belief in a client's innate potential for self-directed growth, regardless of age, and (c) that the concept of self is a continuous process. Utilizing art, sand tray, drama, storytelling, games, and other experiential activities, the client is encouraged to express and make meaning of their internal emotions. This translates into a nondirective, relational, phenomenological exploration of the client's embodied way of being in the world. The capacity to play at any stage of life maximizes our ability to learn new things. Play helps us work through problem areas in our lives that we may otherwise avoid because they are too painful. It enlivens our journey and teaches us to transform states of personal disorder into creative order. Play infuses self-discovery with lightness, and it lends an element of excitement and adventure—even pleasure—to what can be a painful, serious path.

HPT believes that learning and playing are inextricably linked from the earliest stages of life through mother and baby bonding in the form of smiles, tickles, and baby talk. Neuroscience research now supports the theory that this type of interaction between mother and child helps to develop the social brain connections in the infant. Playfulness occurs within relationships, and while it is possible to be playful alone, we have to have experienced it first with another being. The capacity to play is such an important developmental stage that observations of inhibitions in play can be used as a diagnostic tool when assessing children's emotional, psychological, and cognitive development. Research suggests that children who have not been introduced to playful interactions and shared humor will struggle making connections with people in later life and are more likely to approach new situations with higher levels of anxiety.

HPT practitioners distinguish between different types of play: body, object, rough and tumble, spectator, ritual, and imaginative play; all providing specific stimulus to the brain to enhance neural development in children. In HPT the therapist is able to utilize all of these different types of play within the therapy process in order to support the developmental process. Imagination and fantasy naturally form the basis of many types of play in children, from dueling pirates to finger painting, or princess tea party to super hero rescues, the more embodied the process, the more enlivened the play.

Within this framework, HPT and the HERD model of EFP can be visualized as different branches of the same tree, sharing the same philosophical roots. They both stem from a phenomenological, noninterpretative, and experiential process that unfolds in the here-and-now. Combined with the development of a more grounded sense of self in relation through an embodied therapeutic relationship, a child's capacity for self-actualization can emerge. The healing relationship focus shifts in the HERD model to that between the client, horse, and therapist. HPT and the HERD model also share the concept of I-Thou relating, emphasizing interconnectedness and dialogue, and is characterized by authentic meeting and the co-creation of a supportive and healing relationship.

The Stretching Song
Hands up high, to the sky
Way down low, touch my toes
Stretch out wide, side to side,
Arms in a muddle,
Give myself a cuddle!

Mary was a 5-year-old client who was referred to me through an outpatient eating disorders clinic. She had started to refuse to eat anything other than mashed potato. Food that was previously appealing to her had become repugnant. Her mother reported that this had also coincided with Mary suffering from severe separation anxiety and she would panic if she were not within sight of her. Mary already had a younger sister and had another sibling on the way. Her mother's pregnancy had been fraught with physical challenges, and she had taken to feeling responsible for her sister and did not want to leave her side either. In our first session, Mary was solemn and quiet in her demeanor. Her breathing seemed shallow and her energy felt fretful as she spent most of the session wringing her hands together. Mary told me that everything else she "ate-ed" made her tummy feel sick and she didn't want to be sick because that would mean she couldn't "look after Mommy." Dietary allergens had been ruled out by various specialists so she had been referred to therapy. Office-based therapies had not worked. Although Mary was quite articulate for her age, she had refused to engage in the sessions and refused to be left with the therapists on her own. Since Mary was such an animal lover, her parents felt that she might respond to equine-facilitated therapy.

Through the assessment process, it became apparent that Mary was reacting to an earlier trauma of witnessing her mother's sudden hospitalization from acute appendicitis, subsequently followed by a series of pregnancy-related issues that had resulted in needing to go to the emergency room. She had taken responsibility for her mother's health and felt that she needed to be by her side at all times to protect her. Due to her panic attacks and separation anxiety, her nervous system was being overwhelmed by the production of cortisol, a stress hormone that impacts on her digestive system, causing her psychosomatic food reactions.

From an HPT perspective, it was important to honor her experiences and support her to find a way to self-regulate. Traditional talk therapists and her parents had tried to rationalize away her fears and reassure her that Mommy was healthy and that there was no need to panic. Mary's existential experience told her otherwise. Cognitive-Behavioral Therapy techniques had left her feeling unheard and she was prone to having tantrums when she was told she had nothing to worry about. Given this information at the outset, I was keen to support Mary's embodied experience. From the HERD model perspective, it was important to allow her to experience her bodily sensations without them overwhelming her.

From her first session Mary had picked Spirit, a small grey pony mare, to work with. She very quickly became attached to Spirit, grooming her, feeding her, and taking care of her. We worked with Spirit mostly at liberty in the paddock or the round pen so that Mary could witness the freedom of choice that Spirit had. It was important to engage Mary in a way that felt organic to her, allowing her to lead the way toward connecting with Spirit.

Unlike traditional talking therapies held indoors, EFP provides an additional benefit of being held outdoors where the whole environment can become part of the play therapy process. With a creative attitude and the imagination of childhood, anything could become a toy, game, or part of the story. Mary initiated games of follow the leader or finger painting on the horse, and sometimes would ask to sit under a tree to share an apple and tell Spirit stories; all stories centered on the theme of being lost and found. In return, Spirit was very gentle with Mary, and walked with her around the paddock side-by-side or stood quietly under the tree. As with HPT, with each game or story told, the therapist's role is to acknowledge the child's experience and the emotions that surface, while allowing them to make meaning from that experience for themselves. This experiential integration of the meaning that the child makes is at the heart of the HERD model of EFP. Rather than focusing on the cognitive learning to articulate the meaning and broadened awareness in her own process, it was important to allow Mary to sink deeper into herself to find her own agency. In this way, Mary began to grow in confidence that the world around her was a safer place.

As Mary's sense of self developed in relation to Spirit and me, she became more trusting of her own ability to self-regulate and began to initiate more daring play, including asking to ride.

"Miss Veronica, please can we sing that stretching song?" said Mary as she clambered up onto the mounting block in the riding arena. To bring Mary's attention back into her body, I had introduced the stretching song as a prelude to any mounted activity with the horses. The rhyme incorporates a full range of body movements and deep breaths that act as a fun warm up, engaging Mary to become aware of her physical sense of self, as well as acting as a metaphor for growth potential (i.e. how learning anything new is about stretching oneself).

One of Mary's favorite games was to sit bareback on Spirit and finger paint her by stretching forward, backward, and down to every part of the horse that she could reach. With each dab of paint, I encouraged Mary to pay attention to Spirit's reactions. Mary was incredibly detailed in her descriptions of the mare's responses and highly attuned to any shifts in the horse's demeanor. Mary delighted in Spirit turning her head toward her when she was painting, and took this to be a sign that they were playing the game together. This game developed into incorporating the challenge of turning around to sit on Spirit backward and stretching toward her tail. This was difficult for Mary as it involved trusting that Spirit would keep her safe. We spent several sessions imagining sitting backward, and Mary would giggle at the idea of it. When she eventually felt confident enough to turn around, she was thrilled that she was strong enough, and big enough, to reach over Spirit's rump to touch her tail. From that point on, I noticed a shift in Mary's embodied way of being. Her breathing was less shallow; she carried herself more upright; and she moved with much more intention. I wanted to support her embodied experience of this shift and suggested playing with various movements and postures while on horseback.

Mary experimented with lying down on her back to "sunbathe" on the pony, as well as lying "tummy down" to hug her friend. This was an adaptation of the stretching song into a game that incorporated her full body awareness as she began to self-regulate her feelings of anxiety when experiencing anything new. During her play, Mary often commented on how good Spirit was by looking after her and not letting her fall, with each of these observations solidifying her growing confidence that the world around her was a safe place.

Over the course of 20 sessions, Mary was noticeably less tense in her body and had started eating a wider range of foods. She no longer had panic attacks when separated from her mother and sister, although she still experienced a low level of anxiety. While we began with her mother being within sight of her during sessions, now she was tolerant of being dropped off and picked up. By the time we ended our work together, Mary was no longer refusing to go to school and was beginning to make friends. The breathing and stretching games had been incorporated into her everyday life by her own choosing; the stretching song was part of her morning routine that she taught the whole family to sing. By engaging Mary through sight, sound, smell, taste, and feel in the games we played and stories told, she was more able to let go of the anxiety of looking after her mother, and rediscovered her playfulness.

This case study shows how the blending of the key concepts within the HERD model of EFP and HPT result in an integrated modality for working with children. The connections between the HERD model and HPT can be found in their philosophical framework of viewing the self as an embodied, relational process, and the belief in the importance of play and experimentation not only within the therapeutic encounter, but also as a developmental opportunity. Both approaches place the quality of the therapeutic relationship at the center of the healing process and trust that the child is able to self-direct their own growth and learning through a phenomenological and embodied experience of playing, thus providing a supportive developmental environment for the child.

CASE STUDY 6: SINKING INTO SUPPORT

Matthew came into therapy because he was struggling in his relationships with family and friends. He said that he'd been told by his wife of 25 years that he was too controlling and inflexible; too rigid in the way that he did things, and emotionally shut down. He desperately wanted to connect with his wife, his kids, and his friends, but felt stuck and didn't know how to step out of his patterns of behavior. As an army veteran, Matthew held a strong sense of duty and felt that his responsibility in life was to hold the fort and be strong, be the provider for his family, and a rock for his friends. He knows what he knows and he knows how to get things done in his own way.

At 55-years old, Matthew was a tall, heavy-set man. At 6ft 3, he described himself as a "big mountain of a guy who's seen better days." He told me that he was coming into therapy because he wanted to feel more in his life. This struck me as a courageous step. For someone who has spent his whole life building up walls and protecting others, he was essentially coming to therapy to find his vulnerability.

When Matthew arrived for his initial session, the first thing I noticed was how he carried himself. His head was jutted forward, his jaw clenched, his shoulders were stiff, and his arms were rigid. Everything about him looked uncomfortable in his body. His movements were deliberate and slow, but jerky. He walked with stiff heavy legs.

After the preliminary introductions and going through the HERD Safety Protocol, we had spent some time meeting the herd. When asked who he felt most drawn toward, he immediately chose Shiloh, a big stout paint gelding, and a gentle giant of a horse. He'd spent some time grooming and connecting with Shiloh on the ground before I asked if he'd like to experience getting on. Matthew was worried that he'd be too much for Shiloh. I reassured him that the horse was big and strong enough to support his weight and we prepared to mount by putting a bareback pad on Shiloh.

As he stepped up onto the mounting block, I noticed that his legs were ramrod straight, with no bend in his knee. I watched as he first attempted to lift his leg over, also ramrod straight up to the height of the horse before stopping and putting his leg back down. I asked him what he was experiencing in that moment. "I don't know how to support myself to get up," he said.

I asked him what it would be like to ask for support instead of trying to figure it out for himself. "Yeah, I'm not very good at that" he said, "I feel like I should be able to do it by myself." So we processed a little about how it felt to be offered support and how he might open himself up to accept help.

In the meantime, I could see that the rigidity in his body was preventing him from having enough spring in his legs to allow him to get on. "Help" in this instance was getting feedback on how to bend his supporting knee to give him some flexibility to do something new and different for him. I told him what I was noticing and we practiced bending at the knee and softening his hips in order to swing his leg over. The metaphor was not lost on him. "I guess I need help to be more flexible in my life in general," he said.

Once he got on Shiloh, he immediately tensed up in his whole body. "I notice you're holding your breath." He nods, and slowly begins to exhale. The horse, in the meantime, had responded to Matthew's rigid posture by planting his feet and lifting his back up to meet him. I asked Matthew how he was feeling. "I'm ok," he said as he clenched his jaws. I could see that he was perched atop his horse, clothes peg style, with a stiffened lower back and was tilting forward. He commented that he was finding it difficult to find his balance. He made the connection between the physical act of finding balance and his struggle with finding balance in his life.

I explained a little about equitation and the search for a balanced seat. I wondered if finding an embodied sense of balance while on horseback would allow him to integrate that sensation into his life. So I asked if he'd be open to experimenting a little with his posture and he agreed. So we played around a little with sitting back on his pockets and opening his hips a little to bring his lower legs back. With each movement, we checked-in with his breathing and paid attention to any emotions that came up for him. As he sat back, his shoulders came back and he lifted his chin. "Oh, this isn't what I expected at all" he said. "The more I let go, the safer I feel. And it's weird because he doesn't have to stand still like this. He could move and throw me off quite easily."

"So what's it like for you to know that he is willingly supporting you right now?" I asked.

At this, Matthew took a sharp inhale and tears filled his eyes. "I can let go," he said quietly as the tears rolled down his cheeks. "I can feel his strength under me. I mean, I'm a big guy. But it's like I'm no big deal for him to carry. To hold. And I'm so high up, but it's like I can feel the ground beneath me through him."

I let this experience sink in and watched as he exhaled. As he did, Shiloh did too. "I think he's relieved too," said Matthew, and laughed.

I asked if he wanted to try walking a few steps on Shiloh. "Allow him to move you as he walks" I said, mindful of the metaphor in that invitation. We walked about twenty strides, paying attention to his new body posture and his breath. Matthew exhaled deeply and Shiloh stopped. "He moved me," he whispered as the tears rolled once more.

We continued the session with Matthew lying down and hugging Shiloh's neck. I encouraged him to release the tension in his lower back and shoulders, and to allow Shiloh to support him. I watched as he slowly sank deeper into the support that Shiloh offered as he continued to cry.

Matthew explained that he grew up in a military family where it was not acceptable to show vulnerability. As an Army veteran himself, he felt that he had been conditioned to swallow down any uncomfortable feelings, needs, and desires. "Getting the job done right" was the priority. Matthew pointed out that it had been a very long time since anyone was able to physically hold him completely. For him, women and children are the ones who are held. He is always the one that does the holding. For Matthew, the experience of Shiloh's openness to connection, willingness to be present, and his capacity to hold him was a profound one.

This session was pivotal in Matthew's therapy journey. It allowed him to release physically and emotionally some of his rigidity that was stopping him from connecting with the people in his life. Finding his vulnerability, and allowing himself to be moved, physically and emotionally, brought awareness of his capacity for doing things differently. He became more mindful of allowing others to support him and let go of his belief that he always had to be the strong one carrying everyone else; that he deserved to be held and supported as well. The session helped him to begin to release his expectations of himself as needing to be the rock for everyone else, deepen his connections with those around him, offering him the opportunity to be more authentic in his way of being in the world, and support him to come home to his embodied self.

This case study highlights the impact that mounted work can have for clients needing an embodied sensation of support. The physicality of Shiloh supporting Matthew was a profound experience for him. In Shiloh's willingness to stand still while he practiced swinging his leg and mounting, Matthew was also able to see that support was readily available and not something that he had to fight for, or feel he was too much to handle. This embodied experience allowed Matthew to integrate this into his life with a sense of relief, enabling him to bring himself into to contact with others more fully and authentically.

CASE STUDY 7: WE ARE ALL CONNECTED

Working with groups within an EFP setting can pose additional challenges. There are already many variables that are beyond one's control when horses are added to the mix in a therapeutic setting, and group work provides even more unknowns. Whether the group is a closed one for a set duration, or an ongoing open group with shifting membership, maintaining confidentiality and boundaries is of utmost importance. It is something that we prioritize at The HERD Institute and emphasize at the beginning of each group. What happens in the group, stays in the group.

During a weekly therapy group I ran, a participant, Sandy, asked if her husband could join the group for one session. She said he wanted to experience some of the magic that she had told him about. Understandably, the rest of the group members were unhappy with the request, and became concerned about issues of confidentiality. Participants started firing questions rapidly in her direction. How much detail had she been divulging to her husband? Had she mentioned people's names? Did she not respect their boundaries to ask if he could join the group? How could she possibly bring this request into the group?

We were standing out in the paddock with the herd when Sandy brought up her request. It was the beginning of the session on a gorgeous summer day. Sandy had been in the therapy group for about a year, and my experience of her was of someone who was very clear about her boundaries (sometimes to the extreme of being rigid), so was surprised by her request. I knew that she had been struggling in her marriage, and that was part of the reason she had joined this therapy group. I also knew that she was a breast cancer survivor, and had recently been for her annual screening. As the energy of the group began to rise with anxiety, I invited everyone to take a moment to breathe and find their center. I did the same.

As we breathed, the herd walked over and surrounded the group. Infinity, a senior bay Morgan mare, came and stood beside Sandy. I asked Sandy to tell the group more about what had prompted her request. She shook her head and looked down at the ground. Infinity nudged her arm with her muzzle and she turned to look at the mare. Quietly, she told the group that she feared her cancer was back. Her check-up had revealed a small tumor in her lymph node and she was awaiting the results of the biopsy. She had thought that by bringing her husband, who was a professional photographer, to the group for one session, he would be able to take some pictures of her with the horses during the session. She believed that these would sustain her should she need to drop out of the group for medical treatment. Sandy apologized for her clumsy request and for not being upfront about the reasons, saying that it all felt too raw to process yet. While a few of the group members challenged her on that, Sandy was reluctant to process her news further.

Instead, the group discussed what it would mean to allow Sandy's husband to join for one session. Most of the members were in favor of supporting Sandy's request. One participant was concerned that agreeing to this would open the door for others to bring their partners, and wanted the group to agree that this would not set precedence. They agreed to allow Ted, Sandy's husband, to attend the following session, but were clear with their boundaries that he could not take photographs of anyone who was not willing to sign a photo release for him.

The following week, Sandy and Ted arrived. As always, we began with the HERD Safety Protocol, and I reiterated the importance of confidentiality. Ted began by stating that he understood that this was an unusual situation, and he wanted to reassure the group that he was there purely to take photos of Sandy and the horses. Sandy was adamant that she did not become the center of attention in the session simply because Ted was present.

As the group checked-in, the same mare as the previous week, Infinity, came and stood next to Sandy. This was not a horse that she had previously partnered with. Indeed, Infinity would often avoid contact with clients during group sessions, and stand by herself on the far side of the paddock. The group members had often commented on how lonely she looked, and had imagined that she needed comfort. A long-term group member, Charlotte, pointed this out and wondered aloud what brought the mare over. As she spoke, she walked toward the mare. Infinity turned abruptly and trotted away. Charlotte laughed, "She's acting just like you, Sandy. Running away from what she needs."

Infinity turned and walked back to Sandy. I asked her what she made of the mare's actions and of Charlotte's comment.

| Sandy: | I think Charlotte's right. And I think Infinity is telling me that I need to address what's going on. If she's willing to work with me, I guess it's the most genuine invitation I'm going to get. |
| Me: | Well, it doesn't look like she's going anywhere right now. |

Sandy turned to the mare and walked toward her belly. Leaning belly to belly with the mare, she draped her arms over her back and leant into her. Infinity stayed still and exhaled deeply. A few of the group members commented that they had never seen Infinity behave this way before. I turned my attention to Sandy and asked her to describe what was happening for her. Sandy took a deep breath and started to cry. She said she was feeling terrified of what might happen if her biopsy result came back with a malignant diagnosis. If her cancer had returned and was in her lymph nodes, then she knew that it would be harder to fight. What scared her most wasn't the pain and suffering of the cancer treatment and disease itself, but what would happen to her young son who had just turned 8 years old. She recalled her own fear and grief when her mother died of breast cancer when she was a teenager. The thought of her son going through the same agony was too much to bear. She didn't want him to lose her when he was still so young, and knew that it was out of her control. Her helplessness was paralyzing her and yet she knew that she had to stay strong and positive for his sake.

As Sandy talked, she continued to lean against Infinity, who remained steadfast at her side. With every utterance she would bury her head into Infinity's back to hide her tears. After a while, she looked up and noticed that one member of the group was sobbing. Standing opposite her on the other side of Infinity, Janet had started crying almost immediately after Sandy started speaking. Janet was relatively new to the group and had yet to form a close attachment to another group member. As the oldest member of the group, she had found it difficult to relate to the younger members.

| Sandy: | You see? I didn't want to make anyone else miserable with my stuff. Now you're crying as well. |
| Janet: | I need to cry. You're just helping me get there. |

The two women stood on either side of Infinity. The mare turned and nudged Janet on her elbow. "I think she wants me to come closer," Janet said. "May I?" Sandy nodded and reached her hands over Infinity's back. Janet stepped forward and held Sandy's hands. They looked deeply at each other.

| Janet: | I lost my son to cancer when he was 10 years old. The love and protection you feel for yours reminds me of him, and of my loss. A part of me died with him. I'm probably old enough to be your mother, but if you'll let me, I would like to support you somehow in all this. |

By now, most of the group had tears in their eyes. I was feeling moved and deeply respectful of what we were witnessing between the two women.

Life and death. The inescapable existential truths for all living beings. Such poignant beauty.

> Sandy: Yes. It's hard to feel alive when you lose someone. I'm so, so sorry for your loss, Janet.
>
> Janet: And yet we still have to keep living.
>
> Sandy: I can feel Infinity's every breath. She feels so alive!
>
> Me: Can you allow her to support you to feel your aliveness right now?

Turning to Janet, "I will, if you will!" said Sandy. The two women smiled at each other and the group noticeably exhaled. We spent a couple of minutes checking in with the rest of the group. I looked around to see where Ted was, and noticed that he had walked some distance away and was pointing the camera in our direction. I asked Sandy if she wanted Ted to be part of this moment, to help support her. She declined, saying that she didn't want him to feel even more burdened than she was certain he already did. "Besides, Janet said she'd do it with me."

Sandy was once an accomplished rider and competed in 3 day eventing. She explained that it was the one thing that she would always turn to when she felt depressed. Her mother had been an avid horsewoman all her life, so when she was around horses, it made her feel closer to her mom. It also made her feel alive. She hadn't been on horseback since her initial cancer diagnosis. Now, she wondered if she could be supported to ride bareback on Infinity. This was not a simple task as having had a double mastectomy, followed by complications and a number of surgeries, Sandy suffered from nerve damage and pain in her left hip and leg. She was in constant pain and sometimes required a walking stick to support her to walk.

I asked Sandy who she would like to support her in her riding endeavor. Aside from Janet, I asked her to invite two others from the group, or allow members to volunteer themselves. By now, Ted had returned to within earshot of the group. One member, who was an amateur photographer, asked him if he'd like to join in to support Sandy while she took photos for them. Ted looked at Sandy and said that he would be honored to step in if she wanted him to, but would not be offended if she would rather he didn't. Sandy reached out her hand to him and pulled him into the circle that was forming around Infinity. Sandy said that she didn't want to put anyone in a position where they felt obliged to support her, and asked for another volunteer. One woman, Rachel, who had been in the group with Sandy for over 6 months, stepped up to offer her support.

Drawing on my experience as a therapeutic riding instructor, I wanted to ensure that Sandy was securely positioned when mounted. I explained to the group that I needed one person to lead the horse, and one person on either side of Sandy to steady her when mounted. With halter, lead rope, helmet, and bareback pad at the ready, we made our way over to the round pen. Sandy gave Rachel the task of leading Infinity.

Entering the round pen, the rest of the group positioned themselves around the perimeter. Sandy, Janet, Ted, and Rachel made their way into the middle next to the mounting block. I invited Sandy to lead Infinity around the round pen, paying attention to her breathing and connection with the mare. Since she had been standing for a while and was getting tired, Sandy asked Ted to support her on her left-hand side so that she didn't need to use her walking stick. As they walked around the round pen, Sandy stopped after every few steps to turn and pet the mare and to rebalance herself on Ted's arm. It was a sweet interaction, and I felt a sense of warmth towards them. I noticed how her left leg was more rigid when she walked, and she dragged her foot behind her a little. I made note of this as they returned to the mounting block and prepared to mount. I guessed that she would have trouble putting her full weight on her left leg to swing her right leg over the horse to mount.

Checking with Sandy, I asked if her left leg was able to withstand her body weight. She answered no. Assuming that she would not be able to mount after all, she became tearful. I gently suggested that perhaps we could find a way for the others to support her in getting on the horse, without her having to do it all by herself. I explained that in therapeutic riding lessons, we often have riders who are unable to mount on their own, and that there were techniques available to assist them. I described the process of a crest mount, where the rider is positioned and supported to sit on the horse with both legs to one side. With my help, she could lean back slightly while one person held on to her at her waist, and I could help swing her right leg over the horse's neck. Breathing deeply, Sandy recognized that this would take a lot of trust in those around her. She decided that she wanted Janet to be at her back, and Ted to be on the ground ready to help position her right leg in place once I helped her on.

I invited the group in the middle to find a way to connect with each other and Infinity before we mounted. Turning to the rest of the group at the perimeter, I asked that they pay attention to their own breathing, and what was coming up for them as we progressed with getting Sandy on the horse. Looking back to Sandy, I found them holding hands around Infinity. The mare stood with her head bowed, breathing steadily. They looked around their inner circle to take each other in. Sandy nodded slightly and declared that she was ready.

With Janet and me on the mounting block, and Ted on the ground while Rachel positioned Infinity closer to the mounting block, we gently supported Sandy onto her back. Once she was in place, I asked Rachel to lead Infinity to walk forward a few steps away from the mounting block so that Janet could step in beside Sandy. As Sandy looked down at each of us, she began to weep. "Thank you," she said, "I never thought I would be able to do this again."

I asked if she would like to walk around a little and she nodded. I directed Ted and Janet on how to use their forearm on her thighs to steady her as they walked. As Infinity stepped away, I watched as she swung her hips from side to side, knowing that this would impact Sandy on top of her. After a few minutes of walking around, Sandy's weeping gradually turned into giggling. Her body relaxed, and Infinity's hips swung with more freedom.

> Sandy: I feel alive! I feel young again.
> Ted: You ARE alive, and don't you forget it.
> Janet: You look radiant up there.

Stopping to rebalance herself, Sandy looked at the people around her. "I feel so incredibly blessed right now. I'm going to treasure this moment always." She reached down and stroked Infinity on her neck. "She really took care of me. I could feel her walking so carefully. Thank you, Infinity," she said. Looking at me, Sandy smiled. "The amazing thing is that for the first time in years, my hip doesn't hurt, and I don't have pins and needles in my thigh. The nerve damage left me with a constant prickling feeling in my leg. Now it feels warm and soft." She exhaled deeply and asked if she could lie down on Infinity. I nodded and supported her to lie forward on the mare's neck. Infinity turned her head and sniffed Sandy's arm that was draped on her shoulder. "Hi girl," said Sandy, "Thanks for helping me feel free."

I motioned for the rest of the group to gather around and asked Sandy if she would be open to some feedback from the others. "As long as I can stay here while we do that," she grinned. I asked Sandy to look around the group and make contact with each person. I wanted her to take in the support that she had around her, not just from those who had helped her on the horse, but also the safe space that the group had held for her the entire time she was on. As each person spoke, Sandy continued to stroke Infinity's neck. In a group setting, I ask participants to express what they become aware of for themselves as they observe another member's process. It is not a space to comment on what they think is happening, but a relational process that brings out the interconnectedness of humanity.

One member of the group, Natalie, happened to have a history with Infinity, and had at one point leased her as a lesson horse. She had watched the process unfold between Sandy and Infinity, and had been visibly moved from the beginning. Natalie began to speak with tears running down her face.

> Natalie: I have never seen Infinity so tuned in to anyone before. She was so careful with you. I felt so much joy seeing her open up like that. It was like she was adamant that you work with her right from the beginning. She chose you. But, of course, I guess she gets what you're going through. You know she's a cancer survivor too?

This revelation stunned the group, myself included. I had not known that about this mare. Natalie explained that Infinity had had a tumor removed from her chest about 6 years previously. This would have been around the same time that Sandy was originally diagnosed. The synchronicity of the situation was astounding. Sandy leant down to hug Infinity, "So you had breast cancer too!" she exclaimed.

This session illustrates the importance of holding space for clients and horses to interact organically within a group setting. Allowing the group to decide when and how to hold boundaries provides individual members an opportunity to practice self-regulation and self-care. Allowing our equine partners to choose freely when and how they interact with participants offers the group an authentic relational experience. For Sandy, the photos taken of this session have been an integral part of her recovery process. Her biopsy was confirmed as malignant a few days after the session. She was able to rejoin the group for one more session before taking a break for treatment. The remarkable coincidences within the group of Janet's grief and Infinity's cancer history helped Sandy to hold on to the deep connections that she made with both of them. Knowing that she wasn't alone, and that she had support around her alleviated some of the existential anxiety she felt.

It has been almost 3 years since that session. Sandy has been fighting a valiant battle against the disease. Having been in and out of treatment with additional complications, she is now at-home with her husband and son. She tells me that each day that she is alive brings hope that she is one day closer to being in remission. Her remarkable courage and resilience shines through in her journey, and I feel humbled by having been part of it.

CASE STUDY 8: WORKING WITH VETERANS

By Chris Goodall, LISW-S

Chris Goodall is a HERD Institute Faculty member, and is a licensed independent social work supervisor. Chris works with the Louis Stokes Cleveland DVAMC, working in the Psychosocial Rehabilitation and Recovery Center, where she initiated an equine-facilitated psychotherapy program.

The veterans that come through our program have all been diagnosed with a serious mental illness. This includes major depression, bipolar disorder, schizophrenia, schizoaffective disorder, chronic and functionally impairing anxiety, and chronic post-traumatic stress disorder (PTSD). Much of the work we do with veterans involve a history of trauma, and is not always combat related. It is important to note that the experience of trauma does not always result in PTSD. Exposure to traumatic events can trigger chronic mental illness such as bipolar disorder or schizophrenia. Many veterans also struggle with co-occurring addictions. Often these veterans are in their 50s or 60s and have been in mental health treatment for many years. Others are young, recently home from deployment, and new to treatment and their diagnosis. Coming out to the farm often is more appealing than yet another group or individual office therapy. It can be an open door for a younger individual who does not like the idea of "therapy."

There are some special considerations when working with veterans and military service members, though some of these can be broadened to trauma survivors in general, as well as those with serious mental illness and addictions. Being with horses can produce strong nonverbal reactions in our clients. The triggering of strong thoughts, feelings, and memories can lead to avoidance in those not ready or willing to be with that experience. We have found that preparing the veteran for what they may encounter at the farm prior to arrival can be a key to engaging them.

New clients begin with an orientation to EFP that includes a discussion of what EFP is and is not, watching a video of a session, and discussing emotional safety and the likelihood that strong thoughts, feelings, and memories may occur when they engage with the horses. Having this knowledge ahead of arriving at the farm starts to build a trusting relationship with the veteran. We work mainly in a group format due to time and access needs of the Department of Veterans Affairs. Group EFP work can be challenging and asks for a high level of competence in the practitioners. It is important that anyone working with veterans understand basics of military culture, have a background in working with trauma, and have the ability to pick up on nonverbal signals from the client. The horses become a great asset to the therapy team when it comes to picking up on nonverbal communication. A competent EFP practitioner will take cues from their herd in deciding which way to go with a session, trusting the process, and the energy of the horses.

Working with horses provides an open space for self-discovery because it does not have to be verbalized. The standard trauma processing practices offered to veterans ask them to talk about, or write and read about, their trauma repeatedly over the course of several weeks. While some find these methods helpful, there are others who struggle. Working with horses provides a space for the veteran to process their nonverbal reactions and to move through sensations they will typically avoid. They are able to rebuild trust, safety, power and control, self-esteem, and intimacy in an environment that is less threatening and encourages the needed mindfulness to rebalance these areas often damaged due to trauma. When a person experiences trauma, struggles with psychosis, has a traumatic brain injury, or is otherwise neurologically impaired, the brain loses its ability to flex. The frontal lobe goes offline and much decision-making is done out of habit and/or through the limbic system. The role of therapy at this point is often to address issues related to a lack of flexibility including decreased ability to communicate effectively, isolation, avoidance, and inability to perspective take. Being in the presence of horses seems to turn something on in the human directly related to this process. When in the presence of horses, we find ourselves able to focus more fully and truly be present. Because of their military training, veterans often struggle with being present vs. living in their thoughts.

One of the most significant pieces of awareness that happen during an EFP session is that of being present in the moment. This is often significant for veterans who have been trained to disconnect from their emotions and thus their bodies. The value of learning to be mindful and present is one of the most consistent pieces of feedback we've received from veterans that come out to work with horses. Research is starting to show evidence of increased mindfulness as well. Earles, Vernon and Yetz, determined that mindfulness was increased after completing an EFP protocol in veterans with PTSD.

Horses provide a safe space to practice connection. When we are present, we are able to fully engage with another being. Many of the activities we offer in EFP sessions create a space to encourage this connection and bond. Exercises such as breathing with a horse, and walking or moving with a horse, not only require present moment awareness, but also awareness of self and of the horse. Isolation and disconnecting with supports is often a factor for those recovering from serious mental illness. Learning about healthy connection can motivate increased socialization and seeking out supports in everyday life. We've seen this repeatedly with veterans who come out to the farm. Some start to work on repairing relationships with family, others decide to get involved in community activities, or even to volunteer. Some even make a connection between their past experiences and current struggles that positively impacts their recovery.

We often begin with inviting clients to explore connection from a distance. Veterans are encouraged to approach the horses until they notice a response from the horse. They are then to stop and observe where they are in relation to the horse. Many varied results and life lessons come out of this type of experience. Some do not recognize the early signs of connection from 20 or more feet. Others get distracted by other aspects of their environment. Some realize they do not recognize connection until it is tangible. Yet others wait for the horses to make the first move. All of these reactions are information for the veteran about how they currently connect. Any adjustment made with the horses through guided repetition of the activity can lead to corrective awareness and movement in the ability to connect.

For example, a veteran comes into the arena for the day and is asked to approach the horses and stop when they notice a response from one of the horses. She starts to walk forward and finds herself standing in front of a pile of poop. The veteran just stands there, frozen and completely focused on the poop rather than the horses. When asked, the veteran notes that she can't move toward the horses until she cleans up the poop. She describes the horses as being peaceful and in the moment. All traits she would like to work on, but there is some stuff from her past that keeps drawing her attention. She is aware of a metaphor that is building. She really wants to go over to the horses (who are a good 100 feet away), but feels she needs to clean up the poop first. As a practitioner, I am curious about what would happen if she left the poop and walked to the horses, but I am aware that is where I want the journey to go. I choose instead to ask what she would like to do. We talk a bit about how the poop is keeping her from connecting with the horses and that she would like to move forward. She is given a pick and a bucket and allowed to make the choice to clean up the poop. She cleans up some of it, but not all. The veteran then walks out toward the horses. She walks about halfway, stops and observes, making eye contact with a horse. She then moves closer. She talks about wanting to be more like the horses, she talks about what she needs to do to be able to stand where they are and be more in the moment in her life. All of this happens organically, as a part of her journey and connection with these horses. She is able to extend this learning outside of the arena. She makes choices to attend additional treatment, to engage more with family, and to make changes in her life. She chooses to connect more and avoid less.

As I said previously, most of the work we do is group based. Groups are often mixed in terms of diagnosis, age, and even gender. This mix of experiences can often lead to some level of discomfort at first. A part of the process for many veterans is learning to manage this type of discomfort from without and within. Veteran groups from various programs may participate in four, six, or eight sessions. All of these cohorts start with a similar activity—that of observing and then spending some time going to meet the horses. Often in this session we also introduce the concept of breathing with the horses.

Veterans are encouraged to walk up to a horse and place one hand on the withers and another below the belly and then press their head against the rib cage. They are asked to try to match their breathing to that of the horse. These exercises evolve through the course of the group sessions. They can include having the group learn to walk with a horse as a group, or observing and matching their stride to one of the horses. We will (weather permitting) go for a trail walk (in hand) with the horses. This change of pace can be a key experience for the veterans. During all of this, we try to work with the same horses throughout the cohort. The horses and the veterans start to form relationships and get to know each other. When you introduce new horses in each session, this process has to repeat itself each time and cannot go to a deeper level. When you work with the same horses over and over there is a bond formed, deepening trust in another being, and deepening awareness of self, as one can let go of fear and distrust and allow the process to happen. This also happens among the group members.

Often, in early sessions, the group will be asked to go out and do the activity together, yet they will innately move in their own directions. I allow this to happen, knowing that it is information about where these veterans are in their willingness to work with others to accomplish a task. Often, by the end of the sessions, the group has created some connection and moved at least somewhat toward working with one another. Some of the most powerful work happens during those individual moments with the horses.

For example, I once worked with a veteran who struggled with thoughts that he always needed to be doing something, or fixing a problem, or making himself better, or he would slip into a relapse. He was asked to go out and simply stand next to a horse whom he had been working with in previous sessions and identified with. The veteran struggled not to touch, interact with, or otherwise engage with the horse. He became deeply aware of his discomfort in standing still and identified this as an area he would like to work on in his life. It was the combination of being able to touch the present moment, have a 1000 pound being joining with the experience, and being given the opportunity to practice feeling the discomfort of being still that helped this veteran move to his next step in personal development.

Another theme that often arises is that of increased awareness of the effort required to remain focused and in the moment. There is a great deal of mental effort involved in remaining focused on a task, especially when you struggle with racing or intrusive thoughts. Veterans remark on how they didn't realize just how focused they needed to be in order to accomplish a task until they attempted to walk with a horse. Having a benchmark for the amount of effort and type of focus needed for successful movement can now be transferred to other goals or accomplishments in their life.

All of these examples highlight the power of experiencing and being, rather than simply sitting and talking. We have seen veterans who have been in treatment for 20 years come to one equine-facilitated session, and identify issues they have not previously discussed in all those years of treatment. Veterans with chronic pain issues have come out and left their cane on the rail, noting that they are not in pain for the first time in a long time. The horse-human connection is a very powerful bond. I am honored to be able to help bring that connection to our veterans.

CONCLUSION

Each of the case studies described in this chapter have a special place in my heart. Having worked with hundreds of clients over the years, there are many more examples of the beautiful journeys that I have had the privilege of witnessing. I cherish each memory lovingly, and often find myself wondering how a particular client is doing. Occasionally, I will receive an update via an email or card that warms my heart and spurs me on to continue doing this work. The case studies outlined here are but a glimpse of the powerful impact that the HERD model of EFP can provide. Many of the subtleties are diluted when described in words, as so much of what occurs during a session is nonverbal and embodied. So much goes on in each session that it would easily take up an entire book to describe each case study in all its detail.

In working from an existential-humanistic and Gestalt perspective, I believe strongly that bringing myself authentically into each encounter is the only way to facilitate healing. This calls for a high degree of self-reflection and awareness, and it is for this reason that the training offered at The HERD Institute requires practitioners to complete their own personal therapy work and clinical supervision. This is especially true when we bring additional members into our treatment team, humans and/or animals. It is imperative that practitioners are familiar with the horses that they are working with, and have a solid working relationship with their human partners. In this way of working, being able to trust our co-facilitators is absolutely essential. I am deeply grateful for my many equine partners over the years who have brought themselves willingly and authentically into the process with clients, and whom I trust implicitly.

Chapter 10

The HERD Model of EFL in Action

My experience as a management and organizational trainer preceded that of my therapy training. Having worked with large organizations delivering training to all levels of staff, from senior executives to blue-collar workers, I became bored of the run-of-the-mill training programs in my repertoire. When I started to incorporate horses into my work as a therapist, I realized the huge potential for professional development and learning that could be available. My passion in organizational work is witnessing the transformative effect of the horses on participants. So often, corporate clients arrive at the barn expecting the training to focus on the usual concrete theories around teamwork and leadership. What takes them by surprise is how quickly the training moves into a deeper exploration of personal process and individual growing edges. The same exercise conducted with different teams will provide a unique theme every time. It is this organic and fluid process that makes it an exciting endeavor.

My experience also incorporates working with individuals with special needs. As a certified therapeutic riding instructor, I have been privileged to have worked with some incredible individuals, both old and young, and have gained a thorough understanding of the issues brought about by any physical, cognitive, and/or behavioral challenges. Working within this environment is entirely different to that of the corporate world in many respects, and yet, there are some fundamental commonalities.

Whatever the circumstances of an Equine-Facilitated Learning (EFL) session, the focus is always on relationships. Without relationships, teams would not survive. Without relationships, learning cannot take place. Without relationships, there would be no transfer of skills and experience from the arena into the real world.

This chapter provides a number of case studies to illustrate the HERD Model of EFL in action. While the names and identifying information for each client have been changed to preserve their anonymity, the clients' process remains accurate. This chapter offers the reader a chance to appreciate the wide variety of clients that the HERD Model of EFL can be applied to.

Equine-Facilitated Psychotherapy and Learning. DOI: http://dx.doi.org/10.1016/B978-0-12-812601-1.00010-9

CASE STUDY 1: CREATING A "ME"-SHAPED SPACE

Robert was a senior executive at a multinational corporation. He was looking for an innovative coaching program for his leadership team. We met initially at his office where he explained to me what he was hoping to achieve by offering his first-line managers some individual coaching. After conducting a series of performance analytics, 360-degree feedback, and strength-based profiles for his team, he was clear where each individual's growing edge was. He wanted to get them out of their comfort zone and into an environment where they could not hide their habitual patterns of behavior in order to confront them head-on. He had attended a business luncheon where I had presented, and was intrigued by what an EFL coaching session could offer.

I suggested that the best way to find out if I would be a good fit for his team would be to experience an individual coaching session himself. He readily agreed and scheduled to meet me at the barn the following week. He informed me that this was good timing as he had recently been given some feedback that he wanted some coaching on. His director had commented that he needed to learn how to become more visible in the organization, and Robert wanted to see how the EFL session might help with that.

Robert arrived eager to get started but admitted to feeling intimidated by the horses. After going through the safety protocol, we approached the paddock. I invited him to stay on the outside of the paddock until he felt comfortable enough to enter the herd. Robert leaned against the fence watching the herd. We watched as the horses moved around the paddock; Tess, a big Percheron cross; Spirit, a small gray pony; and Lucinda, a Haflinger pony. Tess was chasing the other two away from a patch of grass in the corner of the paddock; pinning her ears and snaking her head. Each time Lucinda attempted to walk over to stand with her, Tess would chase her off. "I guess she's the boss mare then," said Robert.

As he watched, he asked a lot of questions about the horses; their age, sex, background, etc. I noticed that he was filling the space by searching for information. I asked him what it would be like to not know these details about the horses. He took a moment to consider this and replied that it would make him uncomfortable. I challenged him to hold onto the unknown and see what might emerge.

Taking a deep breath, Robert squared his shoulders and announced that he was ready to enter the paddock. I offered him the opportunity to walk around the paddock to meet and greet the horses in whatever way he would like. Upon entering the paddock, Robert walked into the middle and stopped. The three mares were grazing nearby. Robert looked around him with his feet seemingly frozen to the spot. Lucinda looked up from grazing and began to walk over to him. Still, he didn't move. As the mare got closer, he smiled and reached out his hand to pet her on the neck. I heard him introducing himself to her as if she were a new business acquaintance. "Hi, I'm Robert.

What's your name?" he asked. I remained silent as he began to move his feet and made his way to Lucinda's side, at which point she turned and walked away. In the meantime, Spirit had started making her approach from the other side of the field, and was walking up towards Robert behind him. I called attention to this for the sake of safety in case he wasn't aware of her. Robert spun around to face Spirit, and proceeded to offer the same introduction to her as he had with Lucinda.

Spirit circled around Robert, sniffing him and nuzzling his jacket. He smiled and responded by scratching her neck and withers, all the while chit-chatting with her. "Is that nice?" he asked, "Do you like that?" After a while, Spirit stood still and Robert stood with her, gently stroking her neck. He looked across at me expectantly.

Me: So I see you've met Spirit and Lucinda.
Robert: Yes! Is this one Spirit?
Me: It is. And the first one who came by was Lucinda.
Robert: They're lovely. Spirit's very friendly.
Me: What about Tess, over there? (I pointed across the paddock.)
Robert: She didn't come to say hello so I left her alone.
Me: Would it be unusual for you to approach someone if they didn't approach you first?

Robert's eyes widened in response. He told me that this was precisely why his director had made the comments he had. Although Robert was good at his job, eager to learn, and popular with his team, he struggled to make his presence known to those more senior to him in the organization. Since he had already decided that Tess was the boss in the herd, he had automatically avoided contact with her. Robert was stunned that this process surfaced so quickly for him.

I asked if he would like to try approaching Tess. He agreed but voiced his hesitation. I reassured him that I would be right by his side and that he had the choice at any point to change his mind. He walked in Tess' direction slowly. Each time he got within 10 feet or so of her, Tess would walk away. After about five attempts, he turned to me and shrugged. "I guess she's not interested in me," he said. "I don't want to chase after her either," he added. I asked him if this process resonated for him within his work setting. He paused to consider my question and then nodded. "I guess that's what happens with people I consider senior to me. Authority figures in general. If they've not taken an interest already, I don't try to make a point of getting them to notice me." Robert explained that he was brought up to respect authority figures, do as he's told, and not to draw attention to himself. He hadn't realized that this had stayed with him so much, and he could now see how this might impact him in a work setting. He felt intimidated by the "higher ups" in the organization, even though he was steadily getting promoted through the ranks himself, and would find himself feeling tongue tied around the executive directors. In particular, he struggled with networking events and would often end up spending time with one person he already knew, rather than using these opportunities to expand his connections across the organization. He didn't feel comfortable with pushing himself on others, and found small talk unbearable.

I invited him to experiment with approaching Tess in a way that would feel authentic to him. As we talked, Tess began to move in the direction of the other two mares, pushing her way toward the biggest patch of long grass in the paddock. Robert's jaw stiffened and his brow furrowed. "I don't like it that she does that to them," he said. "I'd like to move her out of the way for them." Taking a halter, he approached Tess and gently, but firmly, put it on her and led her away from the long grass. Lucinda and Spirit immediately returned to where they had been grazing before Tess had moved them on. Robert stood with Tess, holding onto her lead rope, and looked around. I offered him the option of working with her in the round pen, or going for a walk with her. "I'd like to go for a walk," he said.

I briefed him on safety procedures regarding leading a horse, and told him that while we were walking, his task was to stop her from grazing along the trail. We walked out of the paddock and followed the trail around the facility. Tess whinnied loudly as we went out of sight from the rest of the herd. Robert was focused on making sure he was holding the lead rope safely, keeping his feet out of her way, and heading in the right direction. He commented that there was a lot to consider in this simple exercise. "I feel like I want to get to know her, but there's so much else going on that's distracting me."

I suggested that we pause and take a breath and reassess the situation. As Robert breathed in deeply, Tess exhaled. Loosening the lead rope in his grip, Robert moved to stand alongside Tess. She turned her head toward him as he stroked her neck. Robert turned to me. "Now I feel like I've met her properly," he said. We continued on our walk on the trail. Tess led the way, pulling ahead on the lead rope with Robert attempting to keep up. Every few steps, Tess would stop and dip her head to graze. Robert would wait patiently until she was ready to move forward again. Each time this happened, Robert would look at me and shrug.

Robert: I don't think that she'd listen to me anyway, so I'm not even trying to get her to stop.
Me: What gives you that impression?
Robert: Well, she's bigger and stronger for a start! So I feel like I need to do what she wants.
Me: And yet you wanted to move her out of the way for the other two earlier.
Robert: I guess that was different. They needed my help.
Me: How does this relate to your situation at work, I wonder?

Robert smiled. He explained that he was very good at championing others, and that's probably what his team values the most in him. He wasn't as confident in championing his own cause. As he spoke, Tess stopped grazing and stood still. I asked him to tell Tess what he struggled with when dealing with the "higher ups" in the organization, and what he would like to be able to do differently. He told her that he wanted to find a way to fit in better, and to be more confident about what he could bring to the table, rather than just following directions. He told her that he often felt that he was looking for common ground, but felt that his background and experiences were more diverse than most of his colleagues, so he struggled to find a space where he could fit. He wanted more of a leadership role, and knew that he would excel were he given the chance, but felt that much of the current leadership team valued a different style than his. He was more collaborative in his approach, and they were more authoritative. He believed in getting to know his team as individuals, finding out what makes them tick and about their lives outside of work. He had been told that he was too "soft" and too afraid to lay down the rules. He could see that the way he was with Tess was how he was with his team. He wanted to be friends first, and leader second. He expressed frustration that it often felt like in order to get ahead at work; he had to force himself to fit into a model of leadership that he didn't entirely ascribe to.

I invited him to walk with Tess again, this time leading her back into the paddock. I explained that I wanted him to get a sense of himself within the herd, of how he could lead and/or follow that felt consistent within his own values. I was curious about how he might interact with the horses given what he had just described. What would that look like? What might that feel like? How and what does he struggle with when leading or following?

Walking back toward the paddock, Tess began to pull ahead. I asked Robert to pay attention to what he felt was acceptable or not, and if not, what could he do differently. Each time Tess pulled, Robert began to circle her around until she stopped. They would walk a few steps before she pulled him again. He circled back. After a few times, Tess stopped pulling and walked alongside him.

Reentering the paddock, Robert took Tess' halter off. She was now at liberty to go back to the rest of the herd or to graze. She did neither. Robert began to walk around the paddock, and Tess followed him. He stopped, changed directions, and still she followed him. Soon, Lucinda and Spirit walked over. Stepping in behind Tess, they began to follow her. Pretty soon, Robert was leading all three mares at liberty around the paddock. He walked a circle with them, serpentined across the paddock, stopped, changed pace and direction, and still they followed. Eventually coming to a halt in front of me, Robert grinned.

"I know what I need to do now," he said. "I can't be a square peg in a round hole. I need to create a ME shaped space in the organization!"

As we processed his experience of the session, Robert remarked that his "a-ha" moment came as he walked back toward the paddock with Tess.

When she pulled ahead, he thought about trying to restrain her with the lead rope and be more forceful in his manner toward her, but that didn't feel authentic to him. Instead, he thought that by redirecting her energy and continuing their momentum in a circle, Tess would realize that he was still with her, but they would go at his pace rather than hers. He was thrilled that the horses followed him willingly, and that he did not have to make himself bigger and bolder in order for that to happen. He acknowledged that his growing edge was to create space for himself without compromising his values and succumbing to a version of leadership that did not fit with his beliefs. It was also important to him to maintain the welfare of the herd in how he felt he managed the relationships between the mares.

I deeply admired Robert's sense of integrity. It is not easy to maintain a personal style of leadership in the corporate world without falling prey to the competitive, macho mentality that can exist within it. Robert found the session so illuminating that not only did he refer his team for coaching, but also persuaded the human resources department at the company to engage the executive board of directors too. This process led to an organizational cultural shift within the company that introduced the language of shared leadership, collaboration, and herd welfare as reference points for progress.

This case study demonstrates clearly the three stages of the HERD Model of EFP. The meeting stage was characterized by the initial needs analysis prior to the client arriving at the barn. Subsequently, the client was given the opportunity to meet the herd. The focus of the session was relational at its core in every sense; between the client and the horses; between me and the client; and between the horses themselves. This phenomenological way of relating was modeled for the client so that he could make meaning of the situation for himself. The key themes that he drew from the session were impactful precisely because it came from him, and not as an interpretation from me. The session was memorable and applicable to him enough for him to generously share his experiences with his team and others, and inspired him to reach for a more creative approach to leading his team. The integration of his learning was evident in how he processed the session, and his subsequent actions.

As seen in this example, the HERD Model of EFL is a fluid, ever-evolving process that follows the client's figure of interest. While there is some direction provided by the practitioner, it does not necessarily involve a prestructured set of activities. This way of working elicits powerful insights for the client, and allows the practitioner to remain phenomenological in their approach.

This next vignette highlights this emergent process when working with more than one person.

CASE STUDY 2: A BUBBLE OF TWO

Jane and Ellie arrived for their coaching session in a fluster. They had requested an emergency session with me, as there had been a staff crisis at their company. As the owners of an exclusive online boutique, these women were phenomenal entrepreneurs. Highly intelligent, fiercely independent, loyal, and creative, they seemed to have it all. Their business had doubled in revenue in the last 6 months and profits were at a record high. They had been in partnership for 3 years and made a tight knit team, but things had recently started to go awry. I had worked with them on a number of coaching sessions prior to this one.

Two nights before our session, they had dismissed their sales director after discovering that she had been fabricating purchase orders in order to increase her commission. This had resulted in a host of miscommunications between Jane and Ellie as they tried to follow up the orders and coming to a dead end. The sales director had set them up against each other, indicating that one had the information that the other needed, and vice versa, sending them into a spiral of confusion. When they eventually discovered the truth, Jane and Ellie felt betrayed and shocked. Due to the infighting that had preceded the discovery, they requested an emergency session to repair the ruptures in their partnership.

The women arrived in a whirlwind of anger and bewilderment. Still reeling in the shock of their discovery, they spent the first 10 minutes of the session talking rapidly, finishing each other's sentences, and talking over each other. It was a beautiful fall day, and we sat by the pond outside the paddock where the horses were grazing.

Me: What do you need from this session today?
Jane: I need to clear my head, and we need to regroup.
Ellie: Yes, we need to realign ourselves so that we can go back in tomorrow on the same page. I feel like we've had so much going on that's distracted us from our vision and partnership, and we need to go back to basics. Remind us of why we're doing this.
Jane: Exactly. I feel like we're off doing our own things and not knowing where the other person is at. We've been spending our time just firefighting and not been proactive at all.

After reiterating the HERD Safety Protocol, I invited them to enter into the herd. I asked them to pay attention to their own personal space as they went into the paddock to greet the horses. I wanted to observe them moving about the herd together to see how they interacted with each other, or not. Stepping into the paddock, they both veered off in different directions. They went from horse to horse to greet them briefly, never staying long with any particular one before moving onto the next. They crossed each other's paths, acknowledging each other as they did, but did not stop to connect with the other. After a few minutes, I asked them how they were feeling and what they were noticing.

Jane reported that she felt like she had to go around to greet all six horses in record time. She connected this to how she felt when faced with her to do list every day; attempting to get through everything as quickly as possible.

Ellie said she felt very confused as she couldn't distinguish the horses from each other very well, so didn't know who she had met and who she hadn't. This resonated with her in the way she tried to keep check of their customers.

I shared my observations with them regarding their lack of contact with each other, despite declaring at the start their intention to reconnect. They looked at each other in surprise, and quickly looked away. I sensed that there was something that had been left unsaid and wondered aloud whether there was something that they were avoiding saying to each other. There followed a long pause.

Eventually, Ellie spoke. "I feel ashamed about what happened. Like I should've been able to catch it sooner. I feel like I've let Jane down." Jane looked at Ellie intently. "It wasn't your fault," she said gently. "We couldn't have predicted this. I feel like you're so caught up with what could've or should've happened that we can't get to what needs to happen now. I'm frustrated. Not at you, but at the situation we're in. And I'm so mad that this woman has managed to drive a wedge between us!"

Ellie looked up at Jane with tears in her eyes. "Me too! That's what I've been most shattered by. That it was so easy for someone else to come between us. I'm sorry for my part in that, Jane." The two women embraced and for a few moments allowed themselves to shed the tears that they had been holding back from each other. They smiled at each other as they regained their composure.

I invited them to revisit the way they greeted the herd. This time, I challenged them to do it together and to pay attention to how they could negotiate this exercise as partners. Giving them a lead rope, I suggested that they begin by both holding onto the rope as a way of staying connected. I asked them to do this in silence without speaking to one another, and instead to be mindful of the nonverbal communication that was available to them.

The two women eagerly stepped up to the challenge. Holding onto their rope, they began to meander through the herd once more. They started by taking turns to point at a particular horse that they wanted to meet. Walking up to each horse, they would pet him/her for a few minutes before pointing to the next. After meeting all of the horses, they returned to me in the middle of the paddock to debrief. They reported that the exercise was simple enough, and that they had enjoyed doing something that focused on them being together. Taking the lead rope away from them, I invited them to repeat the exercise.

This time, as they ventured back out into the herd, Ellie walked a little behind Jane. This prompted Jane to slow down and turn toward Ellie to motion for her to walk beside her. Once they were side-by-side again, Jane set off. Again, Ellie lagged behind. Meanwhile, Freeman and Isaac, the two geldings in the herd started to make their way toward Ellie. Isaac stopped in front of Ellie, blocking her view of Jane, and Freeman stood behind her. Jane had continued to walk ahead, and was unaware that Ellie was no longer beside her. Meanwhile, Isaac and Freeman were circling around Ellie. Each time she made an attempt to extract herself from them, they would move around and circle her again. Eventually, Jane turned around and took in the scene before her. Walking back toward Ellie, she gestured her surprise, raising her hands up to question what had happened. Ellie shrugged her shoulders and furrowed her brow.

Suddenly, the sky darkened and it began to rain. Starting as a gentle drizzle, it soon picked up into a heavy downpour. The horses continued to circle.

Me: What do you make of your experience right now?
Ellie: This is precisely what's happening in our lives right now, isn't it Jane? We've been standing in the middle of a storm for the last few weeks.
Jane: Yes, and I've not been much help to you in the process.
Me: I guess we have a choice right now. We can either take shelter from the storm, or stand in it.
Jane: Never even occurred to us to take shelter!
Ellie: No. But I think we need to weather the storm.

The rain continued relentlessly. The horses continued to circle around Ellie. We stood in the storm. I asked Jane and Ellie to consider their options in that moment; how might they be able to reestablish their partnership? What might they need in order to weather the storm?

Jane decided that she needed to enter into the middle with Ellie to symbolize that they were in the storm together. She took a breath and dodged past Freeman as he circled around. The women linked arms and stood together. I asked them to pay attention to their joint boundaries, and to get a feel for what it was like to be in it together. They stated that they needed to maintain their boundaries, not just as individuals, but to protect their partnership from being intruded upon by others. Jane felt that Ellie was more attuned to their joint boundaries than she was, and asked her for help to pay attention to any infringements upon them. Ellie agreed, and acknowledged that she also needed help from Jane to not become stuck in the past, so that they could attend to the present moment and what might happen next.

Ellie: We need to pay attention and keep our bubble of two safe.
Jane: Yes! Our bubble of two! I know I might not say it enough, but I so value your presence in my life and to share my passion for this business with.
Ellie: Right back at ya, girl! You are an inspiration. I'm going to do my damnedest not to let anyone come between us like that again. As long as we stand firm together, we can tackle whatever happens next.

As they spoke, Isaac and Freeman stopped circling and walked away. Just as suddenly as it had started, the rain stopped, and the sun came out. The two women looked at each other and laughed. Looking up at the sky, Ellie turned to me and said, "Well, we certainly weathered that storm!" Jane grinned, "You just can't make this stuff up, can you?"

We spent the rest of the session with the two women walking arm in arm through the herd, tracking their sense of the boundaries that held their "bubble of two" together, negotiating the path they could take when obstacles threatened to separate them. Each time a horse approached, they would look to each other to agree a course of action, and rather than allowing the horse to walk between them, they stuck together and either redirected the horse or took a different turn as a coordinated effort.

This case study exemplifies the process of tracking clients in the coaching process in a phenomenological manner, allowing them to meet each other and the horses in a way that supported their needs in each moment. Their aim and purpose for the session was to reestablish their connection, to rebuild trust and confidence in their partnership, and to refocus their efforts within their working alliance. We were able to raise awareness of how to maintain their boundaries, both individually and together, to allow for a realignment of their common purpose and an integration of their learning from the experiential process.

CASE STUDY 3: ANTICIPATING NEEDS

Annie was an Executive Sales Director at a multimillion dollar retail conglomerate looking to find a team-building activity for her staff. The company had recently completed a massive restructure at every level of the organization. Leading up to the Christmas holidays, they had laid off 20,000 people. Morale was at rock bottom and her team was under pressure to meet their sales targets. Due to the restructure, there was a lack of team cohesion and a high level of anxiety. There had been a merging of two sales teams who had previously been in direct competition with each other. Annie wanted to provide her team with a clean slate to move into the New Year, and was looking for a team-building event that would lay the foundations for a fresh start.

My initial contact with Annie was over a telephone conversation where she laid out the history of the team, and provided me with my brief: to bring the team together in a fun and engaging environment. When I asked her if there was anything in particular that she wanted the team to focus on that would support her in her role, she answered that she hoped that the team-building event would provide them the tools on how to anticipate her needs and be more proactive so that she could focus on leading them out of their recent difficulties.

On the day of the training event, Annie arrived with her team of 15 employees, excited and eager to dive into the experience. She had briefed her team that they were attending a team-building event, but had waited until the night before to give them the address of where it would be held. She wanted them to be surprised by the unique environment of the barn, so had simply told them to bring warm clothes and sturdy footwear.

During the introductions and check-in, the team members looked bewildered and uncomfortable. Many of them commented on feeling intimidated by horses, and a few complained about the cold. As always, I had sent out joining instructions to the client a few weeks prior to the training, so I had assumed that they would have been prepared for the event. Instead, I too felt a little blindsided by Annie having kept the nature of the training a secret. Pulling out hand and toe warmers, and checking that everyone knew that hot drinks were available throughout the morning, I hoped to alleviate some of their physical discomfort.

My colleague, Elisabeth (Lis) Crabtree, was in position as my Equine Support Staff for the event. Lis had set up the arena in preparation for our first experiential session for the morning by placing some chairs in the arena behind some fence panels for participants to observe the herd. In hearing people complain about the cold, she had pulled out a few blankets and placed them on the chairs.

After going through the safety protocol, we entered the arena and invited the team to take a seat. They huddled together under the blankets and watched Lis and I lead the horses into the arena. I had given the team the instructions to observe the horses in silence, to pay attention to how the horses interacted with each other, and what stories they might be telling themselves in their own minds.

We let the three horses loose in the arena. Huckleberry, a young quarter horse gelding, immediately ran over to the fence panels and stuck his head over the bars to look at the team. Samson, a big, gentle, Belgian cross-gelding, walked into the middle of the arena and stood still. Infinity, the senior Morgan mare, walked around the edge of the arena and sniffed the ground. The team members were engaged and everyone focused their attention on the horses.

Slowly and deliberately, Samson began to lie down. A few team members gasped and giggled as they watched his big, cumbersome frame descend into the soft sand. He groaned as he rolled onto his back and made several attempts to roll all the way over, without success. Infinity walked over toward him and stood above him watching him. Stretching her neck out, she sniffed his face and nudged him on his shoulder. Samson rolled all the way over, and Infinity stepped out of his way. Several team members giggled. Meanwhile, Huckleberry was pacing back and forth along the fence panels in front of the audience. As Samson made his way back up and shook the dust off himself, Huckleberry took off around the arena in a mad dash. Round and round he went, with his head and tail held high. On his third time around, Infinity moved toward the edge of the arena and blocked his path. He came screeching to a halt, exhaled, and sauntered back toward the fence panels.

Checking in with the group, I asked them what they had noticed the horses doing, what it brought up for them, and whether they resonated with what was going on. Someone reported that they felt elated watching Huckleberry. Someone else said that they thought Infinity was helping Samson roll over when he was struggling. Another team member said that they felt that Infinity was the boss, keeping Huckleberry under control when he was getting over excited. Someone commented that they could relate to Huckleberry's curiosity. Another said that they thought that Huckleberry was feeling anxious.

I shared with them that although the three horses had met and spent time together previously, they were relatively new to each other, having only been in the herd together for a couple of months. "That sounds familiar!" called out one of the participants.

I pointed out that this is what happens when we enter a new situation. As human beings, we are preconditioned to make meaning of our immediate experiences based on our previous experience. The same situation being viewed from all our individual perspectives brings about a wide variety of meanings. So how do we get on the same page as a team? How do we find common ground when our perspectives are so different? I wondered aloud how this impacts the individuals in this new team.

"I guess we need to get to know each other," said one participant. "We need to remember that we're all on the same team now, and not in competition anymore," said another.

Following on from their responses, I offered the team the chance to step into the arena to get to know the horses up close. Lis passed out some grooming brushes and we spent some time supporting the participants as they rotated around the horses to pet, groom, and spend time with them. Although the horses were at liberty, they chose to stay with the participants as they got more comfortable being around them. I encouraged each participant to be mindful of the horses' responses as they interacted with them, and to ask if the story they were telling themselves resonated with what happened in their work setting.

Pretty soon, a theme began to emerge. Team members voiced their hesitation in getting to know the horses. In particular, they felt that Infinity was difficult to connect with, and found her to be rather unpredictable in her responses. Her reactions were more abrupt and the same action would elicit different responses. She was also more restless and while she chose to stay with the group, she didn't stand completely still, heightening the participants' anxiety levels.

Hearing their feedback, Annie laughed. "I think they're describing me!" she exclaimed. Annie explained that due to the pressures of her role, she was constantly being pulled in different directions, resulting in her inability to focus on one person, or situation, for any length of time. Consequently, she felt that she may be experienced by her team as unpredictable, restless, and distracted. Annie recognized that this exacerbated the team's sense of uncertainty and anxiety levels.

As Annie spoke, a few team members exchanged glances and nodded. I felt admiration for Annie in taking ownership of her process and admitting this in front of her team. It took courage and showed trust in her team to reveal her vulnerability. I gave her this feedback that was met with more nodding from several team members. I asked her to look around at her team and breathe in that support.

Given their positive responses to Annie, I offered the team the choice of either continuing to work with all three horses, or collectively picking one horse to work with as a team. After a couple of minutes of discussion, they chose the latter, and decided that they wanted to work with Infinity. This seemed like the natural choice, as Annie's a-ha moment had resonated with most of the team.

Lis led Huckleberry and Samson away, and left Infinity in the middle of the arena. I led the group through a breathing and grounding exercise together before describing the next activity. Splitting the team into two groups, we gave each group a long lead rope. I asked each team to pick a leader, and then they were instructed to hold on to the rope to stay connected. I asked them to begin walking around the arena in silence, paying attention to where Infinity was at all times, and making sure that the lead ropes were not dragging on the ground.

They proceeded to walk around the arena. One group started by walking side-by-side. The other walked in a line following each other. After a couple of minutes, I gave them further instructions. Each time I counted to three, they had to change their pace. One, two, three...change! One, two, three...change!

Both groups began to jog around the arena, making sure that they avoided Infinity and each other. After four times of counting to three and changing pace, both groups were struggling to keep up. I asked them to go back to walking. The next set of instructions was given—each time I counted to three, they had to change pace *and* directions. This resulted in much more confusion and laughter between the groups as they struggled to keep up with each other.

Meanwhile, Infinity was walking around the arena taking turns to follow one group, and then the other. When they changed pace, she would stand still for a moment before picking a group to walk with. One group came face to face with her as they changed directions. Infinity stood in front of them blocking their path. As the group attempted to move around her, she blocked them again. On their third attempt, the group managed to dodge Infinity and continued on their path.

Coming back to the center, I asked them to process their experiences. The group that had been walking side-by-side reported that they found it really difficult to get into any kind of rhythm. They realized half way through the exercise that there was too much rigidity in their configuration, but didn't know if they could change what they were doing. No one in the group had indicated that they wanted to, and no one wanted to challenge the leader in the group. The leader, Adam, admitted that he was struggling to get across to the rest of the group what he wanted at each stage, and was frustrated that they didn't seem to understand what he wanted, while also recognizing that he couldn't expect them to read his mind.

The leader in the other group, Karen, empathized with him. She experienced something similar, but had concluded that she wasn't being very clear in communicating what she wanted. She did, however, notice that her team seemed to pay a lot of attention to what the other group was doing, and felt that each time they changed pace, she was being pushed from behind to go faster. Karen translated this to a feeling of competitiveness between the teams.

I asked Karen's group how they felt when they came up to Infinity. "That was hilarious! She kept standing in the way, and we couldn't get past her," said one team member. "I didn't know if we were allowed to push her away, but that's what I wanted to do," said another.

Wrapping up this exercise, I asked the participants to consider the following:

1. When asked to change pace, did anyone consider slowing down?
2. When asked to change direction, did anyone consider backing up?
3. When faced with Infinity, did the group consider stopping?
4. How much awareness did each person have of the others in their team?

So often, when working in this way, participants become so focused on the rules of the activity, and the task at hand that they lose sight of the purpose of the activity. When we translate this learning into a work environment, we can begin to see where a team might become stagnant. Slowing down, backing up, and stopping to reconsider the team's agenda, options, and connectedness is essential for a team to thrive. When processing these questions, the participants can begin to take ownership of their own process and how it impacts on the rest of the team.

Annie was stunned. She had experienced Infinity stepping in front of the group as a direct challenge. The thought of stopping and reevaluating the situation had not occurred to her, and in fact, was the opposite of what she would naturally do. Her instinct was to soldier on and overcome any obstacles in their way. As a saleswoman, this was what she had been trained to do for her whole career. Never take no for an answer. In processing this experience, she recognized that slowing down, backing up, and stopping were valuable options that might allow her to reassess the direction she was leading her team. It would also allow her team to better anticipate her needs.

The final activity of the session aimed to integrate the participants' experiences from the morning. Attaching a lead rope to either side of Infinity's halter, I asked the participants to split into two groups and hold the lead ropes together. Setting up some cones and ground poles in the arena, we created a mini-obstacle course. Asking them to reflect on the feedback from the earlier exercise, I challenged the team to lead Infinity through the obstacle course, weaving the cones and stepping over the ground poles. The focus was on connecting with Infinity and each other to complete the course in silence and in a synchronized manner.

Their attempt was messy. A few team members struggled to keep up, and Infinity stopped after every few steps. Pausing the proceedings, I asked them to regroup and focus on what they had learnt. They recognized that they needed a clear plan and direction and rearranged themselves so that Annie was next to Infinity on one side, and Adam (as Annie's second in command) was on the other. Annie and Adam communicated through hand gestures as to which way they would tackle the course, and paid attention to the team members on the ends of the lead ropes who would have to pick up the pace more than the others as they went around the corners of the arena. With this plan in place, the team embarked on their obstacle course once more.

Their second attempt was better, but still a little uncoordinated. Infinity kept stopping and attempted to turn around mid-way through the course. I asked them what needed to change in order for Infinity to follow more willingly. "We need to make her feel more a part of the team," said one participant. "She needs to feel like we're doing this with her and not just ordering her around," said another. They decided to return to petting her and connecting with her a little before asking her to walk with them. When they were ready, I threw in the final challenge. Removing the lead ropes, I asked them to complete the course with Infinity at liberty.

The participants looked at Annie. She took a deep breath and rallied her troops by offering some positive encouragement, "We can do this guys," she said. "We just need to stick together and take it one step at a time and modify the plan a little." She indicated that she would count them down with her fingers to proceed, and hold her hand up to pause before stepping over each ground pole. The team got into position with Infinity in the middle and set off.

Infinity followed their lead around the cones. Approaching the ground poles, she stopped. Annie held up her hand and the entire team came to a halt. She looked around at the team members on her side and motioned for them to step back a little. They, in turn, looked across at the members on Adam's side to check that they were in line with each other. Adam looked at Annie and nodded to indicate that he was ready. Annie looked at Infinity, counted down with her fingers and they moved on over the poles, coming to a halt back at the start of the cones.

The team was elated at having completed the task. In the feedback session that followed, they indicated that Annie's clear directions and focused attention on each individual member helped them to know that they were on the right track. Adam commented that he felt more able to support Annie and could anticipate what she needed. The team felt that spending the additional time with Infinity allowed her to feel part of the process, much like they do when they are given specific attention and guidance.

This entire session lasted 3 hours. During that time, the participants went from being competitors to allies; from disconnected and anxious, to relational and grounded. Annie was able to give clearer, more precise directions, and focused her attention on what was happening in the moment, rather than being distracted by external pressures, and provided a more coherent framework for her team to follow. In doing this, they were able to anticipate her needs more clearly, and she felt more supported.

This case study illustrates how the HERD Model of EFL can offer a layered experience for participants. The three stages of meeting, relating, and integrating can be clearly identified throughout the process. Beginning with a focus on connection with self, then with others, and then operating from a bigger picture to integrate their previous learning, participants came away with insight into their own process, and a heightened awareness of how small shifts in perspective can impact the success of the team.

CASE STUDY 4: EVERYONE WANTS TO BELONG

Jessica was the Executive Director of a nonprofit organization working with refugee families. The organization aimed to help transition families to their adopted country, and offered psychosocial educational events. One of the programs was a teens group that met once a week to forge friendships with local teenagers in the area. It offered the newly settled participants the opportunity to learn about the culture in their adopted home, and for local teenagers to engage with a culture other than their own. The weekly meetings were facilitated by volunteers from diverse backgrounds and included a retired schoolteacher, a social worker, and a stay-at-home mom. These gatherings varied from restaurant outings, going bowling, attending baseball, hockey, or football games, going to the mall or the movies as well as more structured psycho-educational and psychosocial events. Jessica approached me to conduct an EFL session as a way of introducing the concept of belonging, and to help the group to get to know each other on a deeper level.

In discussing the group's needs with Jessica, we planned a 90-minute EFL session for a group of eight participants. The group would be a mix of newly settled refugees and local teenagers. It was an open group, so attendance varied week to week although alliances had started to form over the past month. Jessica hoped that by offering something in a unique setting would bring more coherence to the group and drive up attendance.

The group arrived on a wet and windy morning. There were five newly settled refugees and three local teenagers, six girls and two boys, all aged between 15 and 18 years old. After the initial introductions and safety protocol, I invited the group to stand outside the gate to the indoor arena where we would be working, while I led the horses into the arena. Cheyenne and

Reba, both quarter horse mares, entered the arena and meandered around. I asked the group to stand at the gate to observe their behaviors in silence, and to pay attention to how they felt while they watched them.

Upon noticing the participants, Cheyenne made her way over to them and stuck her head over the gate to sniff at each person. Reba stood a little way back facing the group but did not approach. Once Cheyenne had greeted everyone, she began to walk away. Reba made her approach toward the gate. Suddenly, Cheyenne spun around and pinned her ears at Reba and trotted back to the gate. Reba turned and retreated. The mares repeated this dance several times, ending with Cheyenne standing lengthways across the gate, blocking the participants' view of Reba entirely.

I asked the group what they made of the horses' interactions. "Cheyenne wants to keep us all to herself," said one girl. "I feel sorry for Reba," said another. "Reba needs to stand up for herself," said one of the boys. "Cheyenne just wants all the attention," said the other, "I think she's jealous," he added.

We spent some time discussing what it meant to want attention and how Reba might be feeling left out and isolated. The emergent theme of belonging didn't take long to surface as some of the group started to talk about their experiences of integrating into their new life. Although their spoken English was heavily accented, they were able to express themselves clearly. One of the local teenagers spoke up, "I know how it feels too. I've felt left out before at school, and girls can be mean and cliquey, and that's why I want to help you guys settle in."

I invited the group to enter into the arena to meet and greet the horses. Bringing out grooming brushes and hoof picks, I showed them how to brush them and pick their feet. The group spent some time with each horse before we circled up to process.

Discussing their experiences of the two mares, the conversation turned toward how to tell who they can trust to be friends. It seemed that friendship felt like a risky endeavor for these teenagers, and yet it was what they yearned for. We talked about the concept of belonging and what that feels like.

As we talked, the horses had meandered in and out of the circle we had formed in the middle of the arena. I asked the group if they had noticed what the horses were doing. One participant said she thought that the horses wanted to be a part of the group. Another said that he thought they wanted to get to know everyone. Someone else commented that she felt that Cheyenne was still trying to chase Reba away from the group. As she spoke, Cheyenne and Reba approached the circle from opposite ends of the arena. Cheyenne pushed her way into the middle of the circle and stood still. Reba nudged her way between two of the participants and stood between them, forming part of the circle.

"See? She just wants ALL the attention," said one of the boys. This was met with laughter from the rest of the group. The girls on either side of Reba were now petting her on her neck. "She's not really getting all the attention though," said one girl, "Reba's actually getting more love by being close to us." The conversation moved on to discussing how sometimes we try to get our needs met in ways that don't serve our purpose. The participants were able to connect how even though Cheyenne appeared to be the center of attention, she may not be getting what she needed, and it was more of an illusion of belonging.

I invited the group to experiment with this embodied sense of belonging, and asked them to walk around the arena and pay attention to who they wanted to stand with, and the distance they wanted to keep. I asked them to include the horses in their awareness. The participants began to walk around in different directions. Some partnered up by walking side-by-side, and others chose to walk alone. Cheyenne and Reba continued to meander around the arena, fading in and out of the group space and occasionally stopping to spend time with someone. After a few minutes, I asked them to continue walking but to collectively think about how they might want to move together as a demonstration of what it feels to belong.

First, they huddled together in the middle. Cheyenne came and stood with them while Reba stayed on the periphery. Then, they began to walk in pairs, linking arms with each other, forming a double line. Cheyenne started to follow behind the final pair in the lineup. Reba started to follow Cheyenne. As they rounded the first corner of the arena, they walked past the barn cat, Carly, who had been sitting in the corner throughout the whole session. As the procession went by, Carly jumped off her perch in the corner and started walking behind Reba.

"Look!" said one participant, "The cat wants to belong too!" Everyone turned to watch Carly trotting behind Reba. The group walked around the arena twice in formation, with Carly bringing up the rear. When they came to a halt, they formed a circle in the middle of the arena once more. Cheyenne, Reba, and Carly, each found a space and stood between participants around the circle.

"This is what belonging feels like," said one of the newly settled refugees, his voice breaking a little. "Welcome home," said his local buddy.

I allowed the poignancy of that moment to sink in with the group. I encouraged them to breathe in the support and belonging that they felt right then so that they could remember this moment and return to it when they felt disconnected back in the real world. At the end of the session, the participants hugged each other warmly and were eager to give treats and cuddles to both the horses and the cat before they left.

This case study illuminates the HERD Model of EFL as a versatile approach for working with a wide range of clients. This session was a memorable one for me as I resonated so much with the participants' struggles to find a sense of belonging. My personal history of displacement was not appropriate to share with them, but I was aware of how much their stories touched me. So it was particularly important that I stayed in a phenomeno-logical framework so as not to interpret the horses' behaviors for the partici-pants, and allow them to make meaning of it for themselves. I was thrilled by Carly's decision to join in the group walk in such an organic way. For me, this was a testament to the participants' authenticity and presence. In their ability to create a feeling of inclusiveness and connection with each other, it even attracted Carly into the group!

CASE STUDY 5: RESILIENCE AND VULNERABILITY

Within the military services, there are programs that offer a range of workshops and family days for their active duty members and families, ranging from fun days out, parenting seminars, and resilience training. I was asked to design and lead an EFL session for one of their family days. The 2-hour session would be a way of engaging military spouses to take part in more workshops and semi-nars, and was designed to offer them a unique experience in personal reflection.

I had recently introduced a new gelding into my herd, so had decided to work with him and my mare Cheyenne in the session. They had been turned out together for about 3 days and seemed to be getting along well, so I had turned them loose in the arena for some herd observation time. There were six participants, one man and five women, and all but one person had never been around horses before. The family day had been an open invitation to local military families, so none of the participants had met each other previ-ously. After going through the safety protocol, I had asked the participants to stand behind the fence panels separating them from the horses. Arrow, my new gelding, had positioned himself in the far corner of the arena away from the group. Cheyenne stayed at the opposite end closer to us. I had asked the participants to observe the herd and notice what stories they were telling themselves about what the horses were doing.

For the first few minutes, the horses paid no attention to each other or the group. Arrow was busy sniffing the ground, and Cheyenne was hovering near the group but not overtly interacting with them. I say "overtly," as I cannot be sure what was going on in her mind, and was not aware of any obvious signals from her of trying to engage us in any way. Her intentions were focused elsewhere. After a few minutes, Cheyenne lifted her head and looked across at Arrow. With an abrupt shift in energy, keeping her sights on Arrow, she began to paw the ground. Suddenly, she pinned her ears and launched herself across the arena toward the gelding. Arrow turned his back on her, showing us his big, powerful back-end. Cheyenne slid to a halt, spun around, and raced back down to our end of the arena. Just as quickly, her energy shifted back to her calm, grounded self.

I looked across at the participants and noticed a couple of them seemed to be holding their breath. I was about to check-in with them when, out of nowhere, Cheyenne pawed the ground in front of her, and repeated her charge. Flying across the arena, she stopped short of Arrow's backside, spun around and cantered back toward us once more. I noticed a couple of raised eyebrows from the group, but decided to wait to see what would emerge before hearing their thoughts. Over the next few minutes, Cheyenne repeated her bull-like charge routine. Eventually, she came back to a halt, exhaled, and shook her whole body.

I turned to the group and asked them to share their experiences. One woman, Sonia, admitted that she was feeling nervous. She had never been around horses before and felt that Cheyenne's energy was quite overwhelming and intimidating. As she spoke, Cheyenne walked in front of the fence panel to where Sonia stood, and began pawing the ground gently. This was different to what she had been doing, and one of the participants commented on it. Slowly, Cheyenne lowered herself onto the ground to roll. The group gasped, as they had never seen a horse do this up close before. Cheyenne rolled onto her back. And there she stayed. Her legs were tucked up in front of her chest, and her back legs were lifted off the ground.

Sonia: I can't believe she's doing that! I was just saying that I felt intimidated by her, and she comes and lies down like a puppy dog, exposing her belly. Like she's saying there's nothing to be scared of, she's just a big softie!"

Upon hearing this, Cheyenne rolled over onto her side, stood up, and shook the dust off in a full body shake. "Just like my dog," said Sonia. I revealed to the group that Arrow and Sonia were relatively new to each other. "Just like us," said Mick, the only guy in the group. "I like that they're getting to know each other, just like we are."

We continued the session with a couple of breathing and movement based exercises in raising awareness of self, other, and environment, which allowed participants to get to know each other more. After conducting a lead-line exercise with all participants holding onto a lead rope to stay connected, the theme of strength and resilience began to emerge. As military families, they were conditioned to respond to situations by staying strong and overcoming obstacles.

I handed out some sticky labels and asked the group to write down words that came to mind when they thought about the need to be resilient. They wrote strength, courage, brave, adaptable, together, bounce back, and fortitude, among others. I invited them to put the sticky labels on the horse that they thought represented these qualities. We stood back and took in the sight of the two horses parading at liberty with these words of resilience on them. I asked the group if there was anything missing. "I guess it doesn't say anything about the actual struggle we're being resilient about," said Maria, the eldest participant in the group.

I agreed, and began to tell them a little about the horses. I explained that even though the group had experienced them as big and powerful, and had attributed all these words of resilience and strength to them, they had their own histories. I revealed that Cheyenne is blind in one eye, and suffers from acute arthritis in both of her hind legs. Arrow, was a rescue from an Amish work farm, and had been retrained as a riding horse. He was adjusting to his new surroundings and still finding his place in the herd. His feet had been badly shod and were rehabilitating, having taken months to regrow, he was only just starting to find his balance. My point was that they were big and powerful, but also susceptible to being highly vulnerable. As prey animals, a horse that cannot see, and a horse that cannot run, would certainly be at risk.

The participants took this information in. One woman began to speak. "I guess it's hard for us to acknowledge our vulnerabilities. We move around so much that it's difficult to know who to turn to. I suppose that's a vulnerability in itself, right?" The others nodded in agreement. The discussion moved on to how to discern support when it is available, and how to ask for it.

Meanwhile, as we talked, Cheyenne had returned to charging at Arrow. Maria watched her, mesmerized by her antics. "This might be too much to share, but I just made a really important connection. I'm watching the horses, and I realized that this is exactly what I do with my husband. I want to connect with him and need his support, but when we're together, I just charge at him with all this anger that's been building up." Her eyes filled with tears. As she wiped them away, Cheyenne walked up to her and stood with her seeing eye facing her.

I thanked Maria for sharing her experience, and that I heard her voice her desire to connect. I pointed out that this was the first time that Cheyenne had engaged one-to-one with anyone in the session, and highlighted that she had her good eye on her. "Maybe she felt my need to connect too," said Maria. I looked around the group and noticed that another woman had started to cry. "I totally resonate with what you just said. Thank you for sharing it with us." Cheyenne moved over to the woman that had just spoken and stayed with her. Each person in the group took turns to speak about how Maria's comments had impacted them, and what they resonated with. As each one spoke, Cheyenne would move and stand with them. The participants all took this to mean that they had been heard, and that Cheyenne was demonstrating that support was available.

Wrapping up the session, I reiterated the importance of allowing ourselves to feel both our strengths and vulnerabilities, and to take away the lesson learnt from the day; that in order to connect with another, it involves taking a risk to sharing our vulnerable parts.

This case study highlights the fine line between EFP and EFL at times. In this session, I was clearly aware of the boundaries and my scope of practice. Were this a therapy session, there would have been so much more to explore with Maria. Given that this was an EFL session, with no therapy remit or support provided, it was important that I acknowledged Maria's contribution, give her time to gather herself, and also weave her story into the learning of the moment. This does not mean that we gloss over the authentic offering from the participant; not does it mean that we linger in it, but find the balance between meeting the participant in what they bring, and providing a safe container for it. Maria's contribution was poignant for the other participants, and provided depth to the session. In line with the HERD Model of EFL, the three stages of meeting, relating, and integrating can be identified throughout the case study. Cheyenne's behavior in this session brought about meaning for the clients from their own phenomenal experiencing, but contained the overarching theme of allowing oneself to show vulnerability while maintaining resilience. Although the client provided the theme of resilience at the beginning, the theme that emerged organically from the group was one of vulnerability and risk. Weaving these threads into the participants' experiential learning allowed them to integrate their experiences into something more concrete for themselves.

CASE STUDY 6: JUST SNIFF

Watching children interact with horses brings an inordinate amount of joy to me. Particularly, children with special needs who are limited in their verbalization skills. The availability for connection that they elicit from the horses never ceases to amaze, and the serenity this engenders in both is always a privilege to witness.

I was invited to design and lead a 12-week program for a middle school extended support services group. Each week, a group of eight students would come to the farm with their teacher and classroom assistants for a 2-hour EFL session. The objective for the program was to provide the students with experiences to enhance their social communication skills, and to learn about teamwork and cooperation. The program was designed to include games and activities that would allow students to interact in an organic manner, giving them space to express themselves in whatever way they needed/wanted to, while providing some boundaries around safety.

The group consisted of 10 and 11 year olds with a wide range of diagnoses, including Downs Syndrome, Autism, Cerebral Palsy, and Developmental Delays. The majority of the students were nonverbal, or had speech delays, and several of them had dual diagnoses of ADHD.

On arrival at the farm on the first week, one student, Markus, immediately caught my attention. He was excited about meeting the horses, and his whole being radiated with joy at this adventure. He smiled broadly and giggled with glee at the thought of being up close and personal with the horses. His enthusiasm was infectious. Markus was 11 years old, and had Downs Syndrome. His intake form suggested that he had difficulty with personal boundaries, and had a tendency to be overly tactile with fellow students and staff members. Although he had good receptive language, his speech was difficult to understand as he struggled to enunciate clearly. Still, he made it clear that he wanted most of all to hug a horse.

After going through our safety protocol, we gathered in the arena. I had chosen to work with Lucinda, a Haflinger pony who I knew was particularly docile with special needs children. She had a wonderful temperament, and would willingly stand to be groomed and petted at liberty patiently. Splitting the group in half, my equine support staff, Zoe, led one group to introduce them to a sticker game of "horse parts," while I led the other group in some grooming. Taking turns to use the curry comb, I led the group in a song about brushing the horse, naming the person who was brushing. Each student was supported to brush the horse, and then hand the curry comb to the next person. While each person brushed, the rest of the group would continue to sing.

Markus loved to sing! He sang loudly and enthusiastically. When it was his turn to brush Lucinda, he indicated that he wanted to hug her. "Later," I said. "First, we brush. Then, we hug," I explained. "Okay," said Markus. "I brush, then hug." So he brushed Lucinda on her neck and then leaned in and kissed her on her shoulder. I was about to comment when he turned his head toward me, still pressed up against Lucinda, who had not moved an inch, and exclaimed, "Oh, she smells good!"

I couldn't help but smile. "Yes, she does smell good, doesn't she?" I replied. Markus grinned and dived back into Lucinda's neck. He breathed deeply and surfaced to exhale, "Mmm. . .just sniff," he said.

Using this as a teaching opportunity, and knowing his difficulties in recognizing boundaries and personal space, I explained to Markus that although Lucinda smells good and she was okay with him sniffing her, it's not advisable to go around sniffing people. I further explained that even if the other person says it's okay, it may not be appropriate. I continued saying that this is the same with hugging and kissing.

Markus looked puzzled for a moment. He looked at Lucinda, glanced back at me, and walked over to the horse's head. "Horsey, I hug you, okay?" he asked. Recognizing this as a step in the right direction, I motioned for him to come and stand by Lucinda's belly. "Put your arm over her back and lean into her belly," I said. "You can hug her this way." Markus did as directed and asked if he could sniff her again. I nodded, and he buried his head into her mane and took a deep breath. "Mm. . .hug and sniff," he said. Lucinda turned her head toward Markus and sniffed him. "She's okay sniffing. She's sniffing me too!" he exclaimed.

After a couple of minutes, Lucinda shifted her weight from one hind leg to the other. I asked Markus to let go of her and she walked away. "Enough sniffing?" he asked. "Enough sniffing," I replied.

Over the course of the next few weeks, Markus developed a ritual when he arrived at the barn. Regardless of which horses we were working with, upon entering the barn aisle, he would make his way over to Lucinda's stall and ask her for a sniff. Sometimes she would stick her head over her gate, and other times she would turn her back. Markus seemed to take these gestures as acceptance or refusal, and react accordingly. It was the beginning of his understanding of personal boundaries.

The rest of the group had all progressed well through the program. Two brothers, who were in foster care after horrendous neglect by their parents, had severe developmental delays. They were discovered by their neighbors at age 6 and 7, after they were heard crying and banging on the door in their apartment. Evidently, they had been abandoned to fend for themselves, and had not been socialized or taught any language skills. As a result, they had developed their own language and were able to converse with each other, and were learning to speak in English. Although their receptive language had developed quickly after they were found, their speech delays were still significant.

One of the boys, Eric, was the class joker. His sense of humor shone through, despite his speech difficulties, and his effervescent spirit was a delight. The other brother, Eddie, was quiet and withdrawn, and other than speaking to Eric in their own way, he would mostly be silent. We discovered, however, that he was motivated to speak to the horses, and so encouraged him to practice his verbal skills by talking to them as he groomed. Eric, on the other hand, needed to work on self-regulation to avoid spinning out of control in a hyperactive state. He was fascinated by my explanation of how to take vitals on the horses in terms of heart rate and respiration, and loved nothing more than to listen to the stethoscope and/or count the horses' breathing patterns. This activity seemed to focus him enough to stay calm and nondisruptive.

In the group activities, the students were encouraged to communicate with each other, working together to achieve a goal. Whether it was leading the horses in the arena in a synchronized pattern, or playing team soccer with the horses (where students kicked the giant soccer ball to the horse at liberty, to see if they would kick it through the goal posts), or taking turns to read a sentence each from a storybook to the horse, the students were supported in their social and communication skills, and increased their awareness of their physical boundaries. Each of these activities was structured with the HERD Model of EFL in mind of meeting, relating, and integrating. Feedback received from post-delivery evaluations for the program included observations from the teacher and assistants of the skills the students were able to transfer from the barn to the classroom. They indicated there was an increase in their ability to self-regulate, focus their attention, and cooperate with classmates.

Working with children with special needs requires the practitioner to connect with students in a different way. In line with our philosophical foundations, the HERD Model of EFL embraces the concept of neurodiversity and is an inclusive approach. Regardless of the cognitive, physical, or emotional challenges that participants face, it is possible to meet them where they are, and work with them to fulfill their potential. It is not an approach that advocates behavior modification, but one that embraces difference by acknowledging that we all process our experiences in our own way. This honors the relational and phenomenological principles at the core of our work.

CONCLUSION

One of the joys of working in this way is that everything becomes part of the process. In the exploration of our own process, and the heightened awareness of self, other, and environment, we can become much more attuned to the world around us. As practitioners, when we begin to practice this way of being-in-the-world, it becomes part of who we are and not just something that we do; we can elicit this attitude in those we teach, coach, train, and work with, and with those in our personal lives. This attitude of abundance and whole-hearted living is at the heart of the HERD approach. It is the belief that if each of us can make a difference in however small a way, these small things add up to big changes; in our families, in our work, in our communities, in our society. This focus on relationship as the bedrock of all learning and healing is infused throughout the philosophy, theory, and practice of the HERD approach, and shines through in each case study presented. In the HERD Model of EFL, the three stages of meeting, relating, and integrating, provide the conditions necessary for the MAGIC of learning to occur.

Of course, none of this would be possible if not for the amazing four-legged co-facilitators we bring into our teams. Our horses, by virtue of bringing themselves authentically into the process, offer participants a level of insight that may not be attainable otherwise. Our relationships with our horses, in terms of the trust we place in them, our belief in their ability to do this work, our knowledge of their skills and limitations, and the trust they place in us to meet their needs, is fundamental to the nature of this approach. For this reason, we must honor their part in the process by treating them with the dignity, respect, and compassion that they deserve.

Part III

Chapter 11

Horse Sense, Business Sense

In addition to a long career as a Business and Management consultant, Elisabeth is an HERD Institute Faculty member and a life-long horsewoman. She is an official coach with the International Society of Rider Biomechanics, a founding member of the International Association of Equestrian Biomechanics, and a Certified Equine First Aid Instructor through Equi-Health Canada.

by Elisabeth Crabtree, MSc, GEP, MIAEB, AISRB

STARTING EQUINE-FACILITATED WORK

As you move from training to practice, you are probably going to start asking yourself how to set up and actually do the work for which you have trained so diligently. For a fortunate few, you may already be employed by an organization that has supported your training and certification. In which case, some of what is discussed in this chapter may not apply. Having said that, this section explores not only the logistics and practicalities required for setting up your own practice, but also discusses your personal readiness in embarking in this work.

SETTING UP SHOP

Setting up an EFP or EFL practice will involve new challenges and opportunities. The purpose of this chapter is to outline some of the considerations that need to be taken into account. For some, the business aspects will be familiar, while the equine components will be new. For others, the reverse may be true. Some topics, such as insurance, licensing, business registration, and legal implications, are highly dependent on where you are located and, for that reason, the guidance provided is intended to be thought-provoking rather than substantive.

Preparing Yourself

Even if you are already working as an established mental health professional, or coach/trainer/educator, you may find it difficult to envisage how your equine-facilitated business is going to look. Accessing programs that offer

Equine-Facilitated Psychotherapy and Learning. DOI: http://dx.doi.org/10.1016/B978-0-12-812601-1.00011-0

guidance and support may be useful and you might want to investigate other practitioners' programs and, where possible, gain first-hand experience. This may include an internship with an EFP or EFL professional—attending conferences, workshops, or seminars offered by existing practitioners and reviewing other professionals' websites.

What Do You Need to Put in Place?

Licensing and/or Registration

Licensing and/or registration requirements vary from country to country and even from state to state. You need to determine what is required for an equine-facilitated professional in your location and proceed accordingly.

Business Entity

You will need to decide on both a business name and the type of business entity that is appropriate: a sole-proprietorship (Assumed Name, DBA, etc.); a limited liability corporation/company (LLC, Ltd, Inc., etc.); or possibly a nonprofit. A limited liability entity offers an extra layer of liability protection. You should seek the advice of applicable professionals (lawyers or accountants) and investigate local, state, and federal tax and registration requirements. When registering a business, the relevant authorities will check to see whether anyone is trading under that business name—so be prepared with an alternative name. Determine in what area (local, national, or international) the business name will be applicable, and research the legal and taxation implications of establishing the business entity.

Once the business entity is established, you can design a logo, purchase a suitable internet domain, and set up a website as well as social media. You need to decide whether you want to create and maintain these sites or invest in professional services. An internet presence is a valuable and important marketing tool. Similarly, you may wish to invest in professionally printed business cards, handouts, and marketing materials.

Accounting

You must also decide how you are going to manage your accounting function. You may have the skills and resources to keep your own accounting records, or you might choose to work with an accounting professional. In either case, you need to keep track of your income and expenditure documentation in order to maintain an accurate set of accounts and prepare tax returns.

Insurance

It is essential to have insurance to cover both your professional liability, as a mental health professional or coach/trainer/educator, and the equine side of your business. If you are working at your own facility, you will also need to have farm and ranch insurance to cover your facility and your horses. There are several companies that offer coverage for equine-facilitated practitioners. If you are working within an existing equestrian facility, you may be able to name each other on each other's policies. If you belong to a professional or equestrian association, you might be eligible for discounts on insurance coverage from certain companies. Be aware of any legislation that offers protection to equine professionals—such as the "Inherent Risk" legislation, which exists in most States in the United States. In many cases, this legislation requires that signs be posted at the equestrian facility, so you may need to invest in some signage in order to gain protection from the legislation.

Liability Waivers and Safety Documentation

You will need to have a Release of Liability signed by everyone at your sessions—both your clients and any assistants or volunteers with whom you work. In some cases, insurance companies either provide templates for this document or require the inclusion of specific wording. In addition, you should have everyone sign a safety agreement in which participants agree to:

- be responsible for their personal safety;
- be responsible for their conduct;
- wear safe and appropriate clothing and footwear at all times;
- wear a suitable, certified riding helmet when mounted; and
- treat horses and humans with respect.

If you are working at a third-party facility, they may have documentation that they also require be signed by all participants, that includes you and your colleagues.

First Aid Training

Equine-Facilitated Psychotherapy and Learning (EFPL) practitioners should be competent in both human and equine first aid before starting the work. Human first aid training is available through many organizations. Equine first aid courses are also available.

You also need to ascertain whether the facilities in which you are going to be working have adequate first aid supplies (both human and equine) and supplement them with your own kit(s), if necessary. You must also ensure that you have access to a phone at all times in case of emergencies.

First Aid Kits

Below are some suggestions for putting together both human and equine first aid kits. In addition, you may want to talk to your veterinarian about any medications and/or wound ointments they might recommend be included, which will depend on where you are located and what your veterinarian prefers that you use.

Taking classes in both human and equine first aid is highly recommended so that you are ready to deal with an emergency.

The quantity of supplies you require will depend on the number of both humans and horses you expect to work with.

HUMAN FIRST AID KIT

Human first aid kits are readily available from a number of retailers and usually contain a good selection of supplies. At a minimum, your kit should contain the following:

Box or bag—labeled "First Aid"
Quantity of nonlatex exam gloves
Antibiotic ointment
Hemostatic granules
Antiseptic cleansing wipes
Hand sanitizer
Sterile dressings—various sizes
Gauze bandages—various sizes
Nonlatex flex bandages
First aid tape
Instant cold compress packs
CPR face mask with one-way valve
Emergency blanket
Triangular bandages
Adhesive bandages—assorted shapes and sizes
Tweezers
Scissors

EQUINE FIRST AID KIT

While some equine first aid kits are available for purchase, you may have to assemble your own. At a minimum, it should include:

Box or bag—labeled "Equine First Aid"
Quantity of nonlatex exam gloves
Veterinary thermometer, with lanyard
Stethoscope
Hoof pick
Shears
Spray bottle
120″ measuring tape
Headlamp flashlight
Hemostatic granules
Poultices

Hand sanitizer
Microfiber towel
Notebook and pencil
Telfa dressings—various sizes
Lubricating gel
Alcohol wipes
Disposable diapers (size 4)
Nonlatex flex bandages
Polo wraps
Cotton roll
Duct tape
Paper towel
Medications recommended and/or supplied by your veterinarian

WHERE ARE YOU GOING TO DO THE WORK?

If you have your own horses on your own property and feel they are suited to the work, you may consider working from home. If not, you may have to investigate the possibility of working at someone else's facility and with other people's horses. Here are some of the factors you need to consider, in either case.

Facilities

There is a wide range of equestrian facilities that may be suitable, for example, therapeutic riding centers, standard riding lesson barns of various disciplines, and existing EFP/EFL barns. Regardless of the type of barn you decide to work in, there are certain criteria you should look for.

The Human-Equine Relationship Continuum

First, and foremost, what type of facility do you feel is a good fit for your personal philosophy? I believe that everyone who interacts with horses sits somewhere on the continuum model, below. Bear in mind that it is a much broader continuum than this illustration would suggest. Spend a moment in introspection and ask yourself where you sit on the continuum. What does that mean for you in terms of being an EFPL practitioner? What are the implications for choosing a barn with which to work? Where might your colleagues, business associates, and clients sit on this continuum?

Horses as commodities
that we can use as we see
fit & treat accordingly

Horses as deities whom
we should impose zero
requirements

2013 ©Elisabeth Crabtree

Finding the right facility may take some time to research. It may involve spending some time, not only at the facility itself, but also with the people who own/manage it to ascertain whether you are comfortable with each other. This applies to both humans and horses. Additionally, consideration must be taken for the following aspects of your chosen facility:

- *Culture and ethics*: Ideally, you will be able to work at a facility offering a supportive atmosphere and positive outlook, where the culture, philosophy, and ideology of the facility are conducive to conducting EFP/EFL. The ethical standards regarding the treatment and husbandry of the horses must be acceptable, and you should be confident in the general standard of horsemanship. You also need to understand the barn rules and feel comfortable working to them.
- *Safety and security*: You should be satisfied with the general standard of maintenance, repair, and cleanliness of the facility and know that safety, emergency, and evacuation plans are in place together with first aid supplies for both humans and horses. You need to feel confident that the facility provides an environment in which you and your clients will be safe, and confidentiality can be maintained, and that you and your clients will be secure. You should determine whether or not there is anyone else on site at all times during your sessions. It is essential that you have access to telephone service at all times, whether via a landline available at the facility, or adequate cell-phone service, in case of emergencies.
- *Cleanliness*: Choose a clean and tidy facility. For many of your clients, this may be their first visit to a barn and they might never have interacted with horses. Their first impressions of the tidiness and cleanliness of the facility will have a major impact on your work. Additionally, a well-kept barn provides a safe and healthy environment for both humans and horses.
- *Logistics*: The facility needs to be located conveniently both for you and for your client population and offer sufficient parking for your needs. You need to consider what workspaces the facility offers for working with the horses (indoor and outdoor arenas, corrals, or round-pens), and whether they are suitable for use year-round in your climate. Additionally, you may wish to have areas for walking around or sitting quietly with your clients during sessions or a meeting room for group gatherings, and there must be adequate restroom facilities. You will probably also want to investigate the available catering options, especially for

group sessions and workshops. Finally, you need to establish whether all areas will be available for use during your sessions. If this is not possible, you will need to establish boundaries regarding noninterruption during your session times within the area that you will be working.

- *Horses*: The barn must have a sufficient number of horses that are suited to the work, and they need to be available at times that are practical in terms of your client population. It is essential that you understand which horses can and cannot be put together, especially for work at liberty. You need to ascertain what tack and equipment is available for you to use, and what you may need to provide.

  - You need to know the horses. If they are your own, you probably already know them well. However, if you are going to work at an external facility, you will need to spend time working with and/or riding the horses that you are planning to partner with. You will need to gain insight into:
    - the horses' temperaments;
    - which horses are suitable for riding (either bareback or under saddle);
    - which horses are only suitable for ground-work with your clients;
    - the idiosyncrasies and habits of each horse;
    - any special considerations or health issues pertaining to individual horses;
    - the herd dynamics, so that you can select horses appropriately for working in groups; and
    - the horses' routines and any other demands on them (riding lessons, therapeutic riding, etc.).

- *People*: You need to find out who else will be at the facility during your sessions, what the implications are for confidentiality and/or interruption during sessions, and whether these can be suitably addressed. It may be that the facility has staff or volunteers who are willing to assist you in the work. If so, you need to establish a working basis on which this is implemented and provide appropriate training. If you are seeking to pursue additional accreditations and certifications, ascertain whether there are people who can provide appropriate assistance and mentorship during the process. Finally, you need to know whether you will have sufficient opportunity to familiarize yourself with the facilities, the horses, and the staff/volunteers at the barn before you start doing the work and you need to be able to negotiate an equitable financial arrangement for using the facility.

Business Arrangements

When approaching potential equine facilities, it is important to think in terms of the value that you will bring to the facility. In addition to any financial benefits you might bring, it may be that you are helping an organization fulfill its mission, or adding a new piece of their puzzle. If you are working with a traditional barn, it may benefit them because your clients (or their families) subsequently decide to take riding lessons, lease or board horses, or put horses into training. For some barn owners, simply being able to help facilitate this type of work may be a reward in itself. Some barn owners have very specific and personal reasons for wanting to encourage this type of work. You need to listen carefully when you meet with them in order to understand the factors influencing their motivation.

You must have a clear idea of how you are going to communicate what you do. This seems obvious but actually explaining EFP/EFL, to someone who has never experienced it, is more difficult than it first appears. Having a list of explanatory and supporting resources that you can either give to prospective partners or direct them to online is particularly useful. These may include articles, research papers, videos, your own and other websites. You also need to explain what you expect from the horses and how you expect the horses to be treated.

You should be very clear that you want to provide a financial benefit for them. If you are charging for your services, you will want to find out the going rate for similar services in your area, set your own rate, and then negotiate an appropriate payment to the barn owner(s). This may be in the form of a percentage or a fixed charge per session. Obviously, this does not apply if you are volunteering your services as part of a charitable therapy barn's provision.

If there is a financial component, you must be very clear on the terms and what you expect in return, discussing rates for both individual and group sessions, and clarifying how many horses may be worked with during each session. Some barns may choose to "sell" their space and horses by the hour/day—be aware that this can become complicated to track. Alternatively, you might establish payment based per session—with individual sessions potentially having access to up to three horses, for example. You might want to be able to work with different horses with different clients (and, in some cases, have the freedom to allow the clients to select the horses—or vice versa), in which case the latter approach is simpler.

An important topic to discuss is the ethics surrounding the work, emphasizing the importance of: (a) confidentiality and (b) freedom from interruption while you are working in sessions. Elicit the barn owner's agreement and cooperation in establishing these priorities with everyone at the barn.

You should discuss timing issues. The time available for you to work may be constrained by other commitments at the barn, such as training or lesson sessions, feeding times, vet and farrier visits, rest days for the horses, horseshows, summer camps, clinics, etc. You must decide whether the times available to you are compatible with the availability of your client population.

Finally, you need to clarify the barn rules and responsibilities, and ask for a written copy if possible. You should obtain written copies of any safety, emergency, and evacuation policies and discuss liability documentation and insurance.

Managing the Space

Once you have found a suitable herd and facility, you should plan to spend enough time to get to know both the space and the horses. Besides becoming familiar with the flow and routines in the barn, you will have the opportunity to deepen your relationship with the barn's owner(s) and connect with their staff, volunteers, and/or clients. This will allow you to become comfortable with the whole facility: the tack and equipment, the arena(s), the stable/stalls, the people, and the horses. Additionally, this is an opportunity to identify any potential issues that may arise. You can identify suitable places for sitting or walking with your clients and clarify that these will be available for you to use. You should take time to explain how and where you want to work with your clients to the barn owner(s) and discuss any issues that arise by maintaining an ongoing dialog.

Advocates

Advocates are the people who really support you in this venture, who encourage you, help you, and talk positively about you to others. Foremost among these are the faculty members, who have been sharing your journey through your training. Others may include family, friends, personal therapists and coaches, and professional colleagues. Keeping your advocates in the loop, regarding all your plans and progress, allows them to help your efforts. Good advocates will help you to network and will themselves expand your networks through referrals. Some may be colleagues willing to provide recommendations or testimonials that you can use in your literature or on your websites.

Clients

Once you have identified the client population(s) with which you want to work, you can start visualizing your ideal client and focus your networking efforts to realize your vision. You should aim to work with a client base with which you are confident, competent, and have the necessary knowledge and expertise.

So, everything is set and you are ready for your first client. Questions you now need to address relate to the practicalities of dealing with clients, such as:

- What releases/waivers/consents, etc. do you need your clients to sign?
- Will the forms be available on your website? Will you email the forms to clients in advance?

- What form will your initial contact with clients take?
- Do you want to offer free first sessions for evaluation?
- How do you expect clients to address you? (children vs. adults? cultural expectations?)
- What kind of atmosphere do you want to establish?
- Where will you initially meet your clients?
- What do you want to explain/show to your clients at your first meeting and what written information, if any, will you hand to your clients (and/ or their parents or guardians, if appropriate)? (these might include appropriate clothing for equestrian work, safety information, barn rules, etc.)
- In a family situation, whom should you include and when?
- How much time will you schedule for each session or workshop?
- How much will you charge (individuals, couples, families, and groups?)
- How much time do you need between clients?

FEE STRUCTURE

Whether you are providing EFP or EFL, what you can charge for your services is hugely dependent on a range of factors: where you are located; what experience and qualifications you offer; whether similar services are available in your area; your client base, and whether you are operating at your own facility or someone else's. You need to evaluate all of these factors, investigate comparable services and decide what is appropriate for you.

NETWORKING AND MARKETING

It is useful to develop a 30-second answer to variations on the question "What do you do?" using nontechnical language and keeping it simple. This allows openings for further questions, and is an important part of the networking process for marketing your business.

How and where you decide to build your networks will depend on your intended client population. Regardless, you should ensure that your advocates know how things are going and with whom you are trying to connect. Joining relevant groups and associations, attending seminars, presenting at networking meetings, and volunteering are all great ways of connecting with people.

Additional considerations might include developing an online presence through your website, Facebook page, and/or other social media. Being able to describe your services in a concise way in laymen's terms will help you to gain traction within the marketplace.

Marketing can become an all-consuming role in itself. You may wish to secure the services of a marketing professional in the first instance to launch your business into the world in an impactful way. This is particularly helpful when you are in the throes of performing due diligence on the other aspects of your business set up prior to launching.

DEMONSTRATIONS AND WORKSHOPS

Once you have a place to work with which you are familiar and comfortable, have established all the necessary boundaries and created a network of interested parties, you can start offering demonstrations and workshops. Additionally, demonstration events can also be a way of showing a prospective barn what you offer. Depending on who wants to attend, you may consider having one event for professionals, and another for those who are simply interested and supportive of your new venture. When arranging events, you need to take into account the number of attendees your facility would be comfortable with, and how many horses would be required.

CONCLUSION

Whether you are starting a private practice, or working within an organization, embarking on this journey of EFPL with clients is both exciting and daunting. There is much to beware of, and there is much to learn along the way. It is essential for practitioners, seasoned, and inexperienced, to hold in their awareness in among the busy-ness of this process, that it is our relationship with our equine partners that is of paramount importance. Without this, the rest of the process cannot unfold. By holding a compassionate and empathic space for our horses, it acts as a model for our clients that this way of being is possible. This translates into the way that we communicate and negotiate with any facilities we might partner with, to offer a mutually beneficial arrangement, and healthy business relationships.

Chapter 12

Final words

This book has offered the reader an introduction to the philosophical and theoretical foundations of an existential-humanistic, and Gestalt approach to Equine-Facilitated Psychotherapy and Learning (EFPL). The Human-Equine Relational Development (HERD) approach to EFPL is deeply rooted in Merleau-Ponty's phenomenology and Buber's I-Thou philosophies. These philosophical concepts have been transposed into the theoretical principles of an embodied relational process and way of being. The HERD models of EFPL outline the steps when working with clients, and are supported by the intricate case studies presented. To aid readers in integrating the philosophy and theory into practice, we offered some practical advice on getting started in an EFPL business. Throughout the book, the issues of ethics and safety are highlighted to ensure that practitioners are aware of what their limitations might be, and to advocate the humane treatment of our equine partners.

In writing a book like this, there is so much that is omitted. The philosophies and theories explored here only scratch the surface of the depth of knowledge that they stem from. There are many resources available for those who wish to delve deeper into the philosophical discussions. Existential-humanistic and Gestalt theories have been extensively explored elsewhere. In the narration of the case studies, the embodied nature of the HERD approach, and the subtleties of movement, gestures, and energetic shifts in both clients and horses, poses a challenge. These limitations aside the philosophies and theories outlined illuminate the healing potential of the HERD approach in practice, and the incredible generosity of our equine partners in their willingness to work with us in this way.

The skills of being a therapist, coach, trainer, or educator cannot be gained from books alone. The art and science of these professions require us to be passionately engaged in the developments in our fields, looking not only to the tried and tested theories, but also to new research and ideas. It also necessitates our commitment to personal and professional development, and the acknowledgment that this is quite often one and the same. Without an awareness of how we bring ourselves into relationships with others, our ways of working may become clouded by our own process. By paying attention to the totality of our phenomenal experience, we support our clients to do the same and make meaning for them. Everything that emerges within an EFPL session is "grist for the mill," contributing to the figures that arise, the

Equine-Facilitated Psychotherapy and Learning. DOI: http://dx.doi.org/10.1016/B978-0-12-812601-1.00012-2

embodied sensations that are elicited, is open for meaning making, and impacts the relational field. It is this creative blend that allows for innovative approaches to emerge, and practitioners are strongly encouraged to look beyond the normative to discover new horizons to immerse themselves in the experiencing of the work for themselves and allow their own style to emerge from it.

Similarly, even with a lifetime of learning to be with horses, one can never stop learning. The more time I spend with my herd, the more I learn from them, the more connected I feel to each of them individually, and collectively. As with psychological and educational theories, there are a multitude of approaches and beliefs on all things equine related. Maintaining an open mind and humility to other approaches allows us to integrate our own experiences and find our own way. While the HERD approach to EFPL is presented here as a clear methodology, it is neither "new" in many respects nor is it the only way. It stems from centuries-old knowledge about being with horses, knowledge that has yet to be quantified but felt on an intuitive and embodied level. It is an invitation to dig deeper within ourselves and our relationships with horses to discover more of what is yet to be revealed. My equine partners on this journey are my greatest teachers. Honoring them with the dignity, compassion, and respect that they deserve is a humbling endeavor in itself. There is so much more to learn, and I encourage each of you to journey with me to come home to relationships with yourself and others, human and equine.

For me, the philosophical and theoretical foundations presented here are not only guidelines for practice, but also are signposts for living, shaping my way of being with all sentient beings through an embodied relational approach. By listening intently to our own desires and honoring our deepest yearnings, we can breathe deeply to allow ourselves to meet, and be met, by another being in the fullness of our authenticity, to broaden our horizons, and reach for our dreams.

There was a time, not so long ago, when I would never have imagined that it would be possible for me to live on a farm, with my herd, to work with clients at my own facility. My wish of creating a training institute was a far-away fantasy. Getting a book published by an academic press was not even on my radar. And yet, life has presented me with my deepest desires. I am blessed and privileged in so many ways, and full of gratitude to all those who have supported me along the way, both two and four-legged.

Reaching for your dreams can be incredibly daunting. The uncertainty of each moment as the process unfolds can create a level of anxiety that feels paralyzing. Yet, when we feel called to follow our hearts and travel off the beaten path, it brings a sense of excitement and adventure. It is this adventurous spirit that many of us can relate to when we decide to embark on this journey of equine-facilitated work. What holds us together is something that is unique to our profession: none of us just fell into it. This isn't a career path that comes by accidentally. Whatever path we took to get here, by the time we reach the point of actually introducing clients to the horses, we have intentionally, passionately, and tenaciously reached for that goal.

It is with this knowledge of our own determination, resilience, and yes, even courage that we are able to meet our clients with conviction, and trust that our horses will help us to facilitate the healing and learning that our clients are seeking. It is with the belief that our own experiences with these majestic, generous-hearted, and noble beings are valid evidence that this way of working can change lives. We bring into each relationship our unique ways-of-being in the world, with curiosity and yearning for relationship. All of this, pointing to our ability to bring ourselves authentically into contact with our clients and horses, is what empowers us to keep doing what we do. Despite the extreme temperatures and hard labor that is often involved when working with horses; despite the sacrifices of money, time, and energy that is inevitable for all horse-owners; despite the heartache that comes when we lose members of our herd; we continue on.

My aim for writing this book is based on my belief in all of that. That our collective wish for those we serve is to find healing through connection with our soulful equine partners. That our collective hope for our industry is that it continues to gain credibility in the wider world. That through introducing people to the wisdom of our herds, we can emulate the authenticity and generosity of spirit that they embody. Through holding an attitude of abundance, we can spread the word to spread the work, and inspire others to follow their dreams.

Bibliography

CHAPTER 2

Bar-on, S., Shapiro, A., & Gendelman, A. (2013). Is animal-assisted psychotherapy a profession? The consolidation of the professional identity of the animal-assisted psychotherapist in Israel. In N. Parish-Plass (Ed.), *Animal-assisted psychotherapy: Theory, issues, and practice* (pp. 297–343). West Lafayette, IN: Purdue University Press.

Cuypers, K., De Ridder, K., & Strandheim, A. (2011). The effect of therapeutic horseback riding on 5 children with attention deficit hyperactivity disorder: A pilot study. *The Journal of Alternative and Complimentary Medicine, 17*(10), 901–908. Available from http://dx.doi.org/10.1089/acm.2010.0547.

Hallberg, L. (2008). *Walking the Way of the Horse: Exploring the Power of the Horse Human Relationship.* USA: iUniverse.

Hamilton, A. (2011). *Zen mind, Zen horse: The science and spirituality of working with horses.* North Adams, MA: Storey.

HeartMath research reference, & Gerkhe, E. K. (2010). The horse-human heart connection: Results of studies using heart rate variability. *NAHRA's Strides, Spring, 2010*, 20–23. Retrieved from http://isar.dk/wp-content/uploads/2012/02/Dr_Kaye_Article.pdf.

Oma, K. A. (2010). Between trust and domination: Social contracts between humans and animals. *World Archaeology, 42*(2), 175–187.

Rector, B. K. (2005). *Adventures in awareness: Learning with the help of horses.* Bloomington, Indiana: AuthorHouse.

Shambo, L. (2013). *The listening heart: The limbic path beyond office therapy.* Chehalis,WA: Human-Equine Alliances for Learning.

Trotter, K. S. (2012). Equine assisted interventions in mental health. In K. S. Trotter (Ed.), *Harnessing the power of equine assisted counseling: Adding animal assisted therapy to your practice* (pp. 1–15). New York, NY: Routledge.

CHAPTER 3

Buber, M. (1965) *Between man and man.* (R.G. Smith, Trans.). New York, NY: Routledge Classics.

Buber, M. (1958). *I and Thou.* (R.G. Smith, Trans.). New York, NY: Charles Scribner & Sons.

Churchill, S. D. (2012). Teaching phenomenology by way of second-person perspectivity (from my thirty years at the University of Dallas). *Indo-Pacific Journal of Phenomenology, 12*(3), 1–14. Available from http://dx.doi.org/10.2989/ipip.2012.12.1.6.114.

King, B. J. (2010). *Being with animals: Why we are obsessed with the furry, scaly, feathered creatures who populate our world.* New York, NY: Doubleday.

Merleau-Ponty M. (2002). *Phenomenology of perceptions.* (C. Smith, Trans.). New York, NY: Routledge. Originally published 1962.

Rowlands, M. (2008). *The philosopher and the wolf: Lessons from the wild on love, death, and happiness.* London, UK: Granta Publications.

Safina, C. (2015). *Beyond words: What animals think and feel.* New York, NY: Henry Holt.

CHAPTER 4

Bugental, J. F. T. (1999). *Psychotherapy isn't what you think: Bringing the psychotherapeutic engagement into the living moment.* Phoenix, AZ: Zeig, Tucker.

Kepner, J. (1987). *Body process: A gestalt approach to working with the body in psychotherapy.* New York, NY: Gardner Press.

Levine, P. (2010). *Waking the tiger: Healing trauma.* Berkeley, CA: North Atlantic Books.

Perls, F. S., Hefferline, R., & Goodman, P. (1977). *Gestalt therapy: Excitement and growth in the human personality.* New York, NY: Bantam Books.

Perls, L. (1992). *Living at the boundary.* New York, NY: Gestalt Journal Press.

Philippson, P. (2001). *Self in relation.* Highland, NY: Gestalt Journal Press.

Polster, E., & Polster, M. (1974). *Gestalt therapy integrated: Contours of theory & practice.* New York, NY: Vintage Books.

Yalom, I. D. (2001). *The gift of therapy: Reflections on being a therapist.* London, England: Piatkus Books. Originally published 1980.

CHAPTER 5

Bachi, K. (2012). Equine-facilitated psychotherapy: The gap between practice and knowledge. *Society & Animals, 20,* 364–380. Available from http://dx.doi.org/10.1163/15685306-12341242.

Hamilton, A. (2011). *Zen mind, Zen horse: The science and spirituality of working with horses.* North Adams, MA: Storey.

Knapp, S. (2013). *More than a mirror: Horses, humans & therapeutic practices.* North Carolina, USA: Horse Sense of the Carolinas Inc.

PATH International (2014). PATH International. Retrieved March 27, 2014 from <http://www.pathintl.org>.

CHAPTER 6

Boylan, J. C., Malley, P. B., & Reilly, E. P. (2001). *Practicum & internship: Textbook and resource guide for counseling and psychotherapy.* Bridgeport, NJ: George H. Bachmann & Company.

Rector, B. K. (2005). *Adventures in awareness: Learning with the help of horses.* Bloomington, Indiana: AuthorHouse.

Schoen, A. S., & Gordon, S. (2015). *The compassionate equestrian: 25 principles to live by when caring for and working with horses.* North Pomfret, Vermont: Trafalgar Square Books.

CHAPTER 7

Buber, M. (1958). *I and Thou.* (R.G. Smith, Trans.). New York, NY: Charles Scribner & Sons.

Bugental, J. F. T. (1999). *Psychotherapy isn't what you think: Bringing the psychotherapeutic engagement into the living moment.* Phoenix, AZ: Zeig, Tucker.

Frank, R. (2001). *Body of Awareness: A somatic and developmental approach to psychotherapy.* Cambridge, MA: Gestalt Press.
Levine, P. (2010). *Waking the tiger: Healing trauma.* Berkeley, CA: North Atlantic Books.
Merleau-Ponty M. (2002). *Phenomenology of perceptions.* (C. Smith, Trans.). New York, NY: Routledge. Originally published 1962.
Ogden, P., Minton, K., & Pain, C. (2006). *Trauma and the body: A sensorimotor approach to psychotherapy.* New York, NY: W.W. Norton & Company.
Philippson, P. (2009). *The emergent self.* London: Karnac Books.
Polster, E., & Polster, M. (1974). *Gestalt therapy integrated: Contours of theory & practice.* New York, NY: Vintage Books.

CHAPTER 8

Kolb, D. A. (2014). *Experiential learning: Experience as the source of learning and development* (2nd ed.). Upper Saddle River, NJ: Pearson Education Inc.
Parent, I. (2016) *Personal communication.*
Perls, F. S., Hefferline, R., & Goodman, P. (1977). *Gestalt therapy: Excitement and growth in the human personality.* New York, NY: Bantam Books.

CHAPTER 9

Bratton, S. C., & Ray, D. (2002). Humanistic play therapy. In D. J. Cain (Ed.), *Humanistic psychotherapies: Handbook of research and practice* (pp. 369–402). Washington, DC: American Psychological Association.
Brown, S. (2008). *Play is more than just fun [Video file].* Retrieved from <https://www.ted.com/talks/stuart_brown_says_play_is_more_than_fun_it_s_vital>.
Duker, M., & Slade, R. (2003). *Anorexia nervosa and bulimia: How to help* (2nd ed.). Buckingham, England: Open University Press.
Earles, J. L., Vernon, L. L., & Yetz, J. P. (2015). Equine-assisted therapy for anxiety and post-traumatic stress symptoms. *Journal of Traumatic Stress, 28*(2), 149–152. Available from http://dx.doi.org/10.1002/jts.21990.
Schneider, K. (2008). *Existential-integrative psychotherapy.* New York, NY: Routledge.

Index

Note: Page number followed by "*f*" refer to figures.

A

AAT. *See* Animal-Assisted Therapy (AAT)
Accounting, 162
ADHD. *See* Attention-Deficit Hyperactivity
    Disorder (ADHD)
Adjuvants, 51–52
Amy's Story, 90–92
Animal life phenomenology, 21
    EFPL and, 22
Animal-Assisted Therapy (AAT), 13
Anorexia nervosa, 92–93, 95–96
Assistants role, 51–52
    adjuvants, 51–52
    cofacilitator, 51
    equine support staff, 51
Attachment process, 101, 109, 113
Attachment theory, 39
Attention-Deficit Hyperactivity Disorder
    (ADHD), 12
Attire, horse safety rules, 50
Authenticity, 24–25, 32–33, 174
Awareness, 28–29

B

Barbara Rector's Adventures in Awareness
    process, 48
Body language, 4
Bracketing process, 30
Buber, Martin, 22–24, 38
    I-Thou, 25–26, 31, 62–63, 65
Business arrangements, 167–169
Business entity, 162

C

Cleanliness, 166
Coaching
    process, 142
    program, 134

Cofacilitator, 51
Cognitive-Behavioral Therapy techniques, 116
Coming home, 67–68
Compassionate Equestrians
    approach, 55–56
    Principles of, 57
Confidentiality, 47, 121
Corporate clients, 133
Criticisms, 85
Culture and ethics, 166

D

DAP system, 50
Deepening, 66–67, 101
Depression, 16, 102
Description, 30

E

EA/FT. *See* Equine-assisted/facilitated therapy
    (EA/FT)
EAE. *See* Equine-assisted education (EAE)
EAGALA model, 15
EAL. *See* Equine-assisted learning (EAL)
EAP. *See* Equine-assisted psychotherapy
    (EAP)
EAT. *See* Equine-assisted therapies (EAT)
Eating disorders, 88
EFL. *See* Equine-facilitated learning (EFL)
EFMHS. *See* Equine-Facilitated Mental
    Health Services (EFMHS)
EFP. *See* Equine-facilitated psychotherapy
    (EFP)
EFPL. *See* Equine-facilitated psychotherapy
    and learning (EFPL)
Embodied relational process, 173
Embodied relational self, 33
Embodiment, 19–22, 32–33
"Energy-in-motion", 39–40

Epistemology, 18
Epoché. *See* Bracketing process
Equalization, 30–31
Equine first aid kit, 164–165
Equine partners, 46–47
Equine support staff, 51
Equine therapy, 10
  EA/FT, 13–14
  EAP/EFP, 14–16
  HERD Institute model
    of EFL, 13
    of EFP, 16
  horses, 8
  therapeutic benefits of human–equine bond
    in, 9–10
  therapy *vs.* therapeutic riding, 10–12
Equine-assisted education (EAE), 14
Equine-assisted learning (EAL), 10, 14
Equine-assisted psychotherapy (EAP), 3,
    14–16
  differing modalities in EFMHS, 14–16
Equine-assisted therapies (EAT), 9–10
Equine-assisted therapy and learning, 9–10
Equine-assisted/facilitated therapy (EA/FT),
    13–14
Equine-facilitated learning (EFL), 3, 10, 133
  EFL practice, setting up, 161–164
  HERD Institute model of, 13
Equine-Facilitated Mental Health Services
    (EFMHS), 14
  differing modalities in, 14–16
    EAP *vs.* EFP, 15–16
    theoretical perspectives and client
      populations, 16
Equine-facilitated psychotherapy (EFP), 3, 10,
    14–16, 61
  differing modalities in EFMHS, 14–16
  EFP practice, setting up, 161–164
  HERD Institute model of, 16
Equine-facilitated psychotherapy and learning
    (EFPL), 3–4, 17, 35, 45, 173. *See also*
    Ethical practice in EFPL
  body language, 4
  community, 37
  horses, 5
  phenomenology and, 21–22
    and animal life phenomenology, 21–22
  practitioners, 163
Equine-facilitated work, 161
Ethical practice in EFPL. *See also* Equine-
    facilitated psychotherapy and learning
    (EFPL)

ethics of working with horses, 55–56
herd safety protocol, 48
horse suitability, 57–59
horsemanship development, 57
leveling playing field, 53–55
professional relationship, 46–48
  client safety, 47
  confidentiality, 47
  continued development, 48
  role of assistants, 51–52
  safe place, 52–53
  safe therapeutic relationship, 50–51
  safety and ethics, 48
  safety around horses, 48–50, 49*f*
Ethics, 48
  and ethics, 166
  of working with horses, 55–56
Evidence-Based Horsemanship, 8–9
Existential humanistic theories, 173
Existential-humanistic psychology approach,
    27–28, 31–32
Experiential learning, 76–79, 153–154
  meeting horses, 78–79

F

Feet (horse safety rules), 49
Felt sense, 33
First aid kits, 163–164
  equine, 164–165
  human, 164
First aid training, 163

G

Gestalt Equine Institute of Rockies, 35–36
Gestalt principles, 97
Gestalt Psychotherapy, 27–28
Gestalt theories, 62–63, 173
Gestalt therapy, 27
Groundwork, 39–40
  working with trauma, 40

H

Heart Rate Variability (HRV), 9
HeartMath Institute, 9
HERD. *See* Human-Equine Relational
    Development (HERD)
"Here-and-now" approach, 28–29
Hippotherapy, 11–12
Holding, 39
Holism, 29–31

Horizontalism, 30–31
Horse sense, business sense
  demonstrations and workshops, 171
  equine first aid kit, 164–165
  equine-facilitated work, 161
  fee structure, 170
  human first aid kit, 164
  networking and marketing, 170–171
  possibility of working, 165
    advocates, 169
    business arrangements, 167–169
    clients, 169–170
    facilities, 165
    human-equine relationship continuum,
      165–167
    managing space, 169
  setting up EFP or EFL practice, 161
  preparation, 161–164
Horse-human interactions, 45
Horsemanship development, 57
Horses, 8, 18, 41, 167, 175
  Buber's *I-THOU* and, 25–26
  ethics of working with, 55–56
  magic, 35–37
  suitability, 57–59
HPT. *See* Humanistic Play Therapy (HPT)
HRV. *See* Heart Rate Variability (HRV)
Human animals, 18–19
Human first aid kit, 164
Human-Equine Relational Development
      (HERD), 3–4, 8, 27, 29, 31, 38,
      40–41, 45, 173. *See also*
      Philosophical foundations
  -based relational instincts, 67
  Institute Codes of Ethics and Professional
      Practice, 45
  Institute model, 37
    of EFL, 13
    of EFP, 16
  meeting, 73–76
    needs of participants, 73–76
    participant, 76
    training/education implementation cycle,
      74f
  Members, 48
  model of EFL, 71–76, 133
    anticipating needs, 142–148
    bubble of two, 138–142
    children interacting with horses, 154
    creating "ME"-shaped space, 134–138
    EFL clients, 71–72
    experiential learning, 76–79

    integrating, 80–81
    nonprofit organization, 148
    relating, 79–80
    resilience and vulnerability, 151–154
    themes, culture, and language, 81–82
    as versatile approach, 150–151
    working with children with special needs,
      156–157
  model of EFP, 61
    Amy's Story, 90–92
    clinical application, 90
    coming home, 67–68
    deepening, 66–67
    embodied touch, 97–102
    first step, 88–90
    Gestalt principles, 97
    habit of picking horses, 86
    integration, 68–70
    integration HPT, 114–118
    language of love, 102–107
    living with anorexia nervosa, 95–96
    members at HERD Institute, 88
    one breath, one movement, 107–114
    release and expand, 63–65, 92–95
    revisiting lessons, 95
    sharing space, 61–63
    sinking into support, 118–121
    space for clients and horses, 127
    value evidence-based, statistical, rational,
      and logical analyses, 87
    working with groups within EFP setting,
      121
    working with veterans, 127–131
  Safety Protocol, 48–50
Human-equine relationship continuum,
      165–167
Human–equine, bond therapeutic benefits of,
      9–10
Human–horse relationship, 8
Humanistic Play Therapy (HPT), 114–118
Hypothetical process, 38

I
I-It, 22–23
  encounter discovering, 26
  modes, 38
  philosophy, 32
"Inherent Risk" legislation, 162–163
Insurance, 162–163
I-Thou, 18, 22–25, 62–63, 173
  connections of phenomenology and, 25

I-Thou (*Continued*)
encounter, 37−38
and horses, 25−26
modes, 38
philosophies, 31, 173
relational approach, 79

L

Leading horses (horse safety rules), 49−50
Liability waivers and safety documentation, 163
Licensing and/or registration, 162
Logistics, 166−167

M

Marketing, 170−171
Memorable, Applicable, Generous, Inspiring and Creative experience (MAGIC), 81
Merleau-Ponty, 19−21, 23, 29
concept, 68
phenomenology, 173
view, 65
Mounted work, 40−42

N

National Guard, 151
Negative emotions, 9
Networking, 170−171
Neuroscience research, 115
Nonverbal communication, 4
North American Riding for the Handicapped Association (NAHRA), 11

O

Ontology, 18

P

PATH. *See* Professional Association of Therapeutic Horsemanship International (PATH)
Phenomenology, 18−22
EFPL and, 21−22
of perception, 19−21
phenomenological method, 29−30
phenomenological relational approach, 79
Philippson, Peter, 31, 65
Philosophical foundations, 17. *See also* Human-Equine Relational Development (HERD)

Buber's *I-THOU*, 22−25
and horses, 25−26
I-It encounter discovering, 26
human animals, 18−19
phenomenology and embodiment, 19−22
philosophical relevance, 17−19
Philosophy, 17−18
Playing field leveling, 53−55
Positive emotions, 9
Post-traumatic stress disorder (PTSD), 127−128
Professional Association of Therapeutic Horsemanship International (PATH), 11
Projection/mirroring, 37−39
"Protective" legislation, 52
Psycho-educational events, 148
Psychoeducational client groups, 74
Psychosocial client groups, 73
Psychosocial events, 148
PTSD. *See* Post-traumatic stress disorder (PTSD)

R

Release and expand, HERD model of EFP, 63−65, 92−95
Resilience, 151−154
Riding, 9

S

Safety, 48
agreement states, 48
around horses, 48−50, 49*f*
safe place, 52−53
safe therapeutic relationship, 50−51
and security, 166
Safety Protocols, HERD, 78, 139
Second-person perspectivity, 22
Self-actualization, 32
Sexual trauma, childhood, 97−98, 101
Sharing space, 61−63, 90−92
Signing liability waivers, 48
SOAP system. *See* Subjective, Objective, Assessment, and Plan system (SOAP system)
Social engagements, 95−96
Somatic Experiencing method, 33
Startle response (horse safety rules), 49
"Strange kinship", 62−63
Subjective, Objective, Assessment, and Plan system (SOAP system), 50

T

Task based client groups, 73
Theoretical foundations, 27–28
  authenticity, 32–33
  awareness, 28–29
  embodied relational self, 33
  embodiment, 32–33
  "here-and-now" approach, 28–29
  holism, 29–31
  I-Thou philosophy, 31
  lost in translation, 32
  "what and how" approach, 29–31
Theoretical foundations II
  attachment, 39
  groundwork, 39–40
  magic of horses, 35–37
  mounted work, 40–42
  projection/mirroring, 37–39
Therapeutic horsemanship, 11–12
Therapeutic interventions, 3
Therapeutic riding, 11–13
  equine therapy *vs.*, 10–12

"Thinspiration", 95–96
Training, 81
Transference in psychotherapy
    literature, 38
Trauma, working with, 40

U

Umwelt theory, 21

V

Verbalization, 48
Veterans, 127–131
Vision (horse safety rules), 49
Vulnerability, 35, 151–154

W

"What and how" approach, 29–31
Workshops, demonstrations and, 171

Printed and bound by CPI Group (UK) Ltd, Croydon, CR0 4YY

08/06/2025

01896868-0009